T0093007

New Technologies in Dermatological Science and Practice

Intelligence, Regeneration, Speed, and Precision

Edited by

Lawrence S. Chan, MD, MHA
Department of Dermatology
University of Illinois College of Medicine
Chicago, IL, USA

M. Peter Marinkovich, MD
Department of Dermatology
Stanford University School of Medicine
Stanford, CA, USA

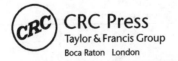

CRC Press
Taylor & Francis Group
Boca Raton   London

CRC Press is an imprint of the
Taylor & Francis Group, an **informa** business

First edition published 2022
by CRC Press
6000 Broken Sound Parkway NW, Suite 300, Boca Raton, FL 33487–2742

and by Taylor & Francis Group
2 Park Square, Milton Park, Abingdon, Oxon, OX14 4RN

© 2022 Taylor & Francis Group, LLC

CRC Press is an imprint of Taylor & Francis Group, LLC

This book contains information obtained from authentic and highly regarded sources. While all reasonable efforts have been made to publish reliable data and information, neither the author[s] nor the publisher can accept any legal responsibility or liability for any errors or omissions that may be made. The publishers wish to make clear that any views or opinions expressed in this book by individual editors, authors or contributors are personal to them and do not necessarily reflect the views/opinions of the publishers. The information or guidance contained in this book is intended for use by medical, scientific or health-care professionals and is provided strictly as a supplement to the medical or other professional's own judgement, their knowledge of the patient's medical history, relevant manufacturer's instructions and the appropriate best practice guidelines. Because of the rapid advances in medical science, any information or advice on dosages, procedures or diagnoses should be independently verified. The reader is strongly urged to consult the relevant national drug formulary and the drug companies' and device or material manufacturers' printed instructions, and their websites, before administering or utilizing any of the drugs, devices or materials mentioned in this book. This book does not indicate whether a particular treatment is appropriate or suitable for a particular individual. Ultimately it is the sole responsibility of the medical professional to make his or her own professional judgements, so as to advise and treat patients appropriately. The authors and publishers have also attempted to trace the copyright holders of all material reproduced in this publication and apologize to copyright holders if permission to publish in this form has not been obtained. If any copyright material has not been acknowledged please write and let us know so we may rectify in any future reprint.

Except as permitted under U.S. Copyright Law, no part of this book may be reprinted, reproduced, transmitted, or utilized in any form by any electronic, mechanical, or other means, now known or hereafter invented, including photocopying, microfilming, and recording, or in any information storage or retrieval system, without written permission from the publishers.

For permission to photocopy or use material electronically from this work, access www.copyright.com or contact the Copyright Clearance Center, Inc. (CCC), 222 Rosewood Drive, Danvers, MA 01923, 978–750–8400. For works that are not available on CCC please contact mpkbookspermissions@tandf.co.uk

Trademark notice: Product or corporate names may be trademarks or registered trademarks and are used only for identification and explanation without intent to infringe.

Library of Congress Cataloging-in-Publication Data

Names: Chan, Lawrence S., editor. | Marinkovich, M. Peter (Matt Peter), editor.
Title: New technologies in dermatological science and practice : intelligence, regeneration, speed, and
    precision / edited by Lawrence S. Chan, M. Peter Marinkovich.
Description: First edition. | Boca Raton : CRC Press, 2021. | Includes bibliographical references and index.
Identifiers: LCCN 2021031157 (print) | LCCN 2021031158 (ebook) | ISBN 9780367639075 (hardback) | ISBN
    9780367639112 (paperback) | ISBN 9781003121275 (ebook)
Subjects: MESH: Skin Diseases | Biotechnology | Artificial Intelligence—ethics | Dermatologic Surgical
    Procedures | Regeneration
Classification: LCC RL71 (print) | LCC RL71 (ebook) | NLM WR 140 | DDC 616.5—dc23
LC record available at https://lccn.loc.gov/2021031157
LC ebook record available at https://lccn.loc.gov/2021031158

ISBN: 978-0-367-63907-5 (hbk)
ISBN: 978-0-367-63911-2 (pbk)
ISBN: 978-1-003-12127-5 (ebk)

DOI: 10.1201/9781003121275

Typeset in Times
by Apex CoVantage, LLC

Contents

Preface

While science and technology have been moving at a very fast speed in the last ten years, and major investments have been placed in artificial intelligence, blockchain technology, 3-D printing, and gene editing, medical practice, including cutaneous medicine (otherwise known as dermatology) is just starting to follow these technology advancements. Moreover, there is currently no published medical textbook of cutaneous medicine that is addressing these particularly needed areas. Enter this book, *New Technologies in Dermatological Science and Practice: Intelligence, Regeneration, Speed, and Precision*. In this book, the frontiers of cutaneous medicine are shown to fill in this knowledge gap. In the first section, "Intelligent Cutaneous Medicine," we devote three chapters to discussing the principles and ethics of artificial intelligence and the utilization of artificial intelligence for clinical imaging and for cutaneous histopathology. In addition, we also include a chapter on a new imaging technology, termed *optical coherence tomography*, as an intelligent method for skin disease diagnosis. In Section II, "Regenerative Cutaneous Medicine," we dedicate the first two chapters to depicting the regeneration of hair and skin utilizing 3-D bioprinting techniques. A third chapter is devoted to the regeneration of skin barrier by eco-friendly approaches. In Section III, "Speed Cutaneous Medicine," we devote one chapter to the utilization of mass spectrometry for intraoperative skin cancer margin detection, with potentially substantial time saving for Mohs micrographic surgery as it is currently performed. Section IV, "Precision Cutaneous Medicine," includes two chapters on precision gene therapy for skin diseases, focusing on treatments for heritable blistering skin diseases. Lastly, a chapter on precision treatment for autoimmune blistering diseases by utilizing CAR-T cells concludes this book. This book is, indeed, a timely intellectual investment for cutaneous medicine.

This book is written for medical educators. It aims to alert medical school faculty members to the need to include these medical advancements in their teaching curriculum. This book is also for dermatology residents as it aims to bring them the up-and-coming technology that may affect their future practices. Importantly, this book is designed for practicing dermatologists, who care for patients with skin diseases on a daily basis. This book aims to provide them with up-to-date information regarding the new cutaneous medicine technology coming their way. Finally, this book is for medical researchers in the area of skin diseases: we hope to inspire them to investigate and generate more novel methodology for the future of cutaneous medicine, in diagnosis and therapy.

Contributors

Peter E. Andersen
Department of Photonics Engineering
Technical University of Denmark
Lyngby, Denmark

Kamran Avanaki
The Richard and Loan Hill
Department of Bioengineering
University of Illinois at Chicago
Chicago, IL, USA

Işın Sinem Bağcı
Department of Dermatology
Stanford University School of Medicine
Stanford, CA, USA

Imogen Brooks
St. John's Institute of Dermatology
Faculty of Life Sciences and Medicine
King's College London, London, UK

Angelina G. Chan
School of Humanities and Sciences
Stanford University
Stanford, CA, USA

Lawrence S. Chan
Department of Dermatology
University of Illinois College of
Medicine and Captain James Lovell
FHCC
North Chicago, IL, USA

John A. M. Dolorito
Department of Dermatology
Stanford University School of Medicine
Stanford, CA, USA

Joanna Jacków
St. John's Institute of Dermatology
Faculty of Life Sciences and Medicine
King's College London, London, UK

M. Peter Marinkovich
Department of Dermatology
Stanford University School of Medicine
Stanford, CA USA

Adam Sheriff
St. John's Institute of Dermatology
Faculty of Life Sciences and Medicine
King's College London, London, UK

Kunju Sridhar
Department of Dermatology
Stanford University School of Medicine
Stanford, CA, USA

Acknowledgments

The editors would like to first thank all the contributors for their dedicated work in making this book possible. We would like to thank our academic institutions, University of Illinois, College of Medicine and Captain James Lovell Federal Health Care Center (Dr. Chan) and Stanford University School of Medicine (Dr. Marinkovich) for their generous support. We would further like to thank our family members for their understandings during our time spent on writing and editing this book.

PART ONE

Intelligent Cutaneous Medicine

Artificial Intelligence

1

Basic Principles and Algorithmic Ethics

Lawrence S. Chan

Contents

DOI: 10.1201/9781003121275-2

3

INTRODUCTION

In this section, "Intelligent Cutaneous Medicine," several clinical applications with artificial intelligence (AI) are described in detail. Thus, there is a need to provide a short introduction to the concept of AI. Not being a computer science expert, I took the responsibility of writing this chapter reluctantly. Using some of my engineering background and having refreshed the mathematical knowledge of which I once had good command during my undergraduate college days, I read several books about it and then drilled into the subject that I am not familiar with. In an odd way, this may turn out to be more suitable for the readers of this book, since I will be using non-jargon language to discuss the topic of AI for the majority of the readers who are also not experts in computer science. Describing what I, a novice, would understand to the non–computer experts will make the subject matter easier to comprehend. Consequently, this chapter is not intended to give an in-depth technical description of AI. Rather, it is an introduction to the concept in a non-technical fashion so that the readers can have a better appreciation of the applications of AI in cutaneous medicine in Chapters 2 and 3.

INTELLIGENCE DEFINED

The term AI implies a special kind of intelligence, although in an artificial manner. Thus, it is proper to first clearly define the term "intelligence" before we define the artificial one. According to the Merriam-Webster Online Dictionary, intelligence is defined as "the ability to learn or understand or to deal with new or trying situations" and "the ability to apply knowledge to manipulate one's environment or to think abstractly as measured by objective criteria (such as tests)" [1]. Similarly, the *Cambridge Dictionary* defines intelligence as "the ability to learn, understand, and make judgements or have opinions that are based on reason" [2]. As stated, the ability to learn, understanding and applying knowledge, a skilled use of reason, and a mental acuteness are implied in intelligence.

AI DEFINED

In terms of AI, the adjective "artificial" is defined as "made by people, often as a copy of something natural" [3] and "humanly contrived often on a natural model: man-made"; "caused or produced by a human, especially social or political agency"; and "lacking in natural or spontaneous quality" [4]. Accordingly, AI implies a man-made type of non-natural intelligence. The main concern of computer scientists is that AI behaves like a person with intelligent behavior; as one computer expert stated: "The goal of AI is to develop machine that behave as though they were intelligent" [5]. A more comprehensive definition of AI has been described by another computer scientist as "computing technologies that resemble processes associated with human intelligence, such as reasoning, learning and adaptation, sensory understanding, and interaction" [6]. Interestingly, some field experts have used a functional term "collaboration" to describe their relationship with AI [7].

A BRIEF HISTORY OF AI

AI has a short but interesting history. Not surprisingly, the Massachusetts Institute of Technology (MIT), an institution with a major focus in science and technology advancements, had a major role in its development right from the start. With its intellectual roots at MIT, the following is a brief, not necessarily comprehensive list of milestone activities in AI development:

- John McCarthy (who joined MIT in 1956) was generally credited as the first scientist to coin the term "artificial intelligence" in 1955, when he organized a 1956 workshop at Dartmouth University in New Hampshire to clarify the concept of a "thinking machine" with a group of researchers in language simulation, neuro networks, and complexity theory [8]. Consequently, the year 1956 is properly considered to be the birth year of AI [5].
- John McCarthy invented the LISP (acronym for list processing, a formal mathematical language) programming in 1958 at MIT [9].
- John McCarthy and Marvin Minsky cofounded the MIT AI lab in 1959 [10].
- The term "machine learning" was coined by the scientist A.L. Samuel in 1959 [11, 12].

- John McCarthy became the founding director of the AI lab at Stanford University in 1965 [13].
- The deep learning network was developed by using principles derived from the general framework of the human neural network in the 1980s [14–17].
- IBM joins force with MIT in 2017 to establish a new MIT-IBM Watson AI lab., with a ten-year, $240 million new investment from IBM. The new lab aims to advance AI hardware, software, and algorithms [18].
- More recently, Dr. Reif, president of MIT, announced major initiative in February 2018 to enhance research in human intelligence and AI in its AI lab, which already has more than 200 independently funded principal researchers [19].

COMMERCIAL INVESTMENT IN AI

Over the last few years, commercial organizations have made substantial investment in the development and acquisition of AI instrumentation and AI applications. On the global level, investment in and spending on AI were estimated to be $35 billion in 2019, increasing by more than 40% from 2018. The level of spending on AI systems is predicted to reach near $80 billion by 2022. The results of AI investment are expected to add a huge $15 trillion to the global economy by 2030. The factors contributing to this growth include worker productivity increase, personalization of product and service improvement, cybersecurity threat prevention and detection, and cost-saving pattern identification. From the perspective of healthcare, AI has the potential to reduce costs by assisting physicians technically and making diagnosis remotely, enhancing disease detection, improving diagnostic accuracy, and optimizing therapeutic effectiveness [20]. Anticipating the substantial impact of AI-driven automation will have on our society and reflecting on the concern of AI-induced job loss by more than 70% of surveyed US citizens, the MIT president has called for decisive actions to foresee and prevent undesirable manpower displacement in a recent op-ed in the *Boston Globe* [21].

BASIC PRINCIPLES OF AI

Having discussed the short history of AI development and the current commercial investment in AI, let us now examine some operational basis of AI.

Deep Learning

Deep learning (DL) is essentially a special type of ML derived in the 1980s to model the working principles of the human neural network. As stated by one expert in the field, "Artificial neural networks are systems motivated by the distributed, massively parallel computation in the brain that enables it to be so successful at complex control and recognition/classification tasks" [24]. Another expert stated it this way: "Artificial neural networks (ANNs) are biologically inspired computer programs designed to simulate the way in which the human brain processes information" [25]. In essence, what the biological neural networks can accomplish is mathematically mimicked (or modeled) by a weighted, directed diagram (or grid) of highly interconnected neurons (or nodes, in AI terms). With the brain being the central command of human intelligence, it is entirely fitting that its nerve network is utilized as the framework of an important aspect of AI. The DL system usually contains multiple layers of artificial neural networks. The neural networks of DL include an input layer, a hidden layer or layers in the middle, and an output layer [14–17]. The "learning" of DL is carried out with input-output samples provided by the training set and by a succession-based algorithm, which adjusts the network weights, such that the network response closely approximates the desired response governed by the training set [24]. It is important to recognize that DL networks accumulate their "knowledge" by detecting the patterns and relationships in the dataset and "learn" from experience, not from programming [25]. A neural network is formed from hundreds of single units of artificial neurons (or nodes, process elements) that are connected with weights (also called coefficients) that are adjustable. Each neuron has weighted input, transferring function, and one output. During the training (or learning), data from training sets reach these neurons and are weighted, and the sum of these weights becomes an activation signal of the neuron and transfers out as an output. The optimization of the accuracy of the output (prediction) is done through adjusting the inter-unit connections and the weights, until the error in prediction is minimized. Once the network is trained (or has learned) and tested, it will have the ability to accurately predict the output when it is given a brand-new input [25]. Figure 1.1 illustrates a simplified graph of a neural network. One scholarly paper succinctly depicted the functionality of DL with this description:

> Deep learning allows computational models that are composed of multiple processing layers to learn representations of data with multiple levels of abstraction. These methods have dramatically improved the state-of-the-art in speech recognition, visual object recognition, object detection and many other domains such as drug discovery and genomics. Deep learning

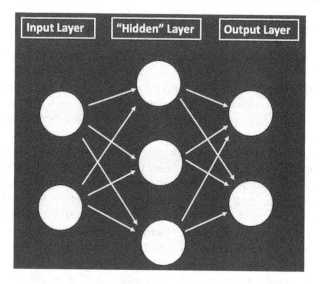

FIGURE 1.1 A simplified diagram of neural network, consisting an input layer, middle hidden layer(s), and an output layer. The information or data flow is one directional, from input to output.

discovers intricate structure in large data sets by using the backpropagation algorithm to indicate how a machine should change its internal parameters that are used to compute the representation in each layer from the representation in the previous layer. Deep convolutional nets have brought about breakthroughs in processing images video, speech and audio, whereas deep recurrent nets have shone light on sequential data such as text and speech [16].

Convolutional Neural Network (CNN)

A CNN processes data that comes in the form of multiple arrays, including one-dimensional signals and sequences, two-dimensional images or audio spectrograms, and three-dimensional video or volumetric images. For data input, such as color images, which are typically in the form of multiple arrays, CNN is usually the preferred choice [16]. As we will see in Chapter 2 (AI in Cutaneous Imaging) and Chapter 3 (AI in Cutaneous Histopathology). where color images are the targets of diagnostic applications, CNN is the preferred AI method.

Recurrent Neural Network (RNN)

For computational tasks involving sequential inputs, such as language and speech, RNN is commonly the preferred choice. RNN processes inputs in a sequential way, one element at a time. Due to the advanced architecture, RNN has been rated very well in predicting the next character in the text or the next word in a sequence [16].

COMMON AI APPLICATIONS IN MEDICINE

As one expert in the field accurately pointed out, the systems offered by AI today are not a universal recipe, but a workshop with a manageable number of tools for very different tasks. Most of these tools are well-developed and are available as finished software libraries, often with convenient user interfaces. The selection of the right tool and its sensible use in each individual case is left to the AI developer or knowledge engineer [5].

Among the many AI applications commonly used in medicine are ML and DL (neural network). The concerns about losing human control notwithstanding, some physicians are hopeful that AI can help bring back the humanity to medicine by reducing the mundane tasks that now require substantial human effort. The many AI applications that are currently applied to or likely will be utilized in medicine commonly include medical diagnosis based on images (or pattern recognition). Medical specialties such as radiology, pathology, ophthalmology, and dermatology will benefit from this category of AI applications. Other areas of medicine that are not pattern based, such as internal medicine, will be able utilize AI in reducing human efforts in performing tasks that can be efficiently handled by machines, such as medical record entering, literature search, automated diagnostic suggestion, lab test recommendation, drug interaction warning, medication error prevention, and antibiotic discovery [26]. Moreover, AI can provide a personalized approach to medicine, assist public health operations, and improve the delivery efficiency of the healthcare systems [27–29]. In addition, medical education, such as simulation-based surgery and medicine training, could benefit from utilizing AI applications [30]. One medical educator envisioned how AI could be applied in medicine this way:

> I am excited about the future, about the power to harness Big Data. By their sheer capacity to plow through huge datasets and to learn as they go along, artificial intelligence and deep learning will bring tremendous precision to diagnosis and prognostication. This isn't to say they will replace

humans: what those technologies will provide is a recommendation, one that is perhaps more accurate than it has ever been, but it will take a savvy, caring, and attentive physician and healthcare team to tailor that recommendation to—and with—the individual seated before them. [31]

AI applications in the dermatology specialty are depicted in the following two chapters.

ALGORITHMIC ETHICS

Although AI is a man-made computational process, it can divert to areas outside our intended purpose, therefore producing undesirable side effects. Two big concerns that challenge academic computer scientists are the issues of fairness and privacy [23]. When it comes to medicine, both of these two concerns are critically important. Since bias in fairness and error leading to privacy breakdown can be introduced by the algorithm of AI application, the ethics of algorithm design and the potential remedies are worthy of our discussion.

Fairness Consideration

Considering the simple actions of data collection and analysis of an AI algorithm, unfairness would be an unlikely outcome of this seemingly level playing field. However, many well-controlled experiments performed online have clearly illustrated the occurrence of political, racial, financial, and gender bias in web-based information services, including major servers like Facebook and Google [23, 32–35].

Privacy Consideration

Along with the great benefit of Big Data, which can be collected and analyzed by AI to benefit us as patients, we also become the data in the process. Thus, our private personal and healthcare information is vulnerable to unintentional exposure. Indeed, there are many documented cases of privacy breakdowns resulting in exposure of sensitive information about specific persons, including their financial data, web search habits, and health records [24, 32, 36]. One excellent example noted by field experts was that while triple data such as zip code, sex, and birth date could not individually reveal a person's identity, combined, they could be used to identify the person. This kind of privacy breakdown was documented by an MIT student who was able to locate such information about the Massachusetts governor, the very person who promised his citizens that they could not be identified by these triple data [23].

Ethical Algorithm Design

Knowing the identified and potential misbehaviors of algorithms, remedies are needed. Some discussions focus on eliminating AI participation in certain areas if the negative long-term consequences outweigh the benefit to the society. Hopefully, most of the problems in AI algorithms are fixable. A recent report from the European Commission High-Level Expert Group on Artificial Intelligence stated the following three sequential framework steps for building trustworthy AI applications [37]:

- Developing ethical principles including respect for human autonomy, prevention of harm, fairness, and explicability.
- Setting requirements to capture ethical perspectives relating human agency and oversight, technical robustness and safety, privacy and data governance, transparency, diversity/non-discrimination/fairness, societal and environmental well-being, and accountability.
- Implementing trustworthy assessment tailored to specific application.

Traditionally, the remedies would be from legal authorities, regulatory agencies, or consumer groups. However, experts in the field have come to realize the inadequacy of these fixes and now instead advocate a new approach, using ethical algorithms to counter such violations. Thus, there is an emerging scientific approach of "socially aware algorithm" design. The aim of this noble ethical algorithm design is to better protect humans from the unintended consequences of poorly designed algorithms while encouraging the beneficial advances of technology. It seems ironic that the field experts who brought the problem of algorithm misbehavior into the society now propose to fix the problem themselves. Nevertheless, the computer scientists who create an algorithm are likely to be the most knowledgeable about the technical details, drawbacks, and limitations essential for the corrective actions, and correcting the mistakes internally may be more effective than having it done by the external forces. Even if ethical algorithms are available, regulatory agencies may need to be involved if search engines choose not to adopt these ethical models for the sake of their engines' accuracy. As we will see in the discussions that follow, developing ethical algorithms will likely come at a price.

Having stated that, one of the biggest challenges for algorithm design to eliminate privacy breakdown and to maximize fairness is how to determine a right balance between the need for accuracy and the concerns of fairness and privacy. Since the key goal of ML is maximum predictive accuracy, this goal could be in conflict with the introduction of new goals of fairness and privacy. The difficult question is whether we can accept an ML algorithm that would be fairer and privacy protective in exchange for a slower search result (like that of Google.com), a less accurate recommendation (like that of Amazon.com), or less efficient traffic navigation (like that of Waze.com). The encouraging fact is that quantity of trade-offs between accuracy and good behavior can be determined, and field experts in these areas of study have suggestions to involve all stakeholders and to consider these values—accuracy on one hand and fairness/privacy on the other hand—on sliding scales when we make decisions on algorithm design, so as to achieve optimal trade-offs between these two sets of values [23].

OTHER UNINTENDED CONSEQUENCES OF AI IN MEDICINE

In addition to the critical issues of privacy and fairness, there are other concerning issues that could result from AI applications in medicine as unintended side effects, both positive and negative [6, 38, 39]:

- Reducing physicians' skills: The overreliance of AI-led automated determination could decrease physicians' abilities to make clinical judgements and decisions in the long term. This could result in detrimental outcomes when the AI machine breaks down.
- Providing out-of-context information: The focus on text (or data) at the expense of context could result in misleading information for physicians.
- Disregarding medicine's intrinsic nature of uncertainty: The tendency of ML to impose an ideal data accuracy and completeness does not take medicine's intrinsic uncertainty into consideration, thus underrating observer variability, leading to a negative impact on ML performance and medical usefulness.
- Changing physician makeup: The revolution of AI driving medical practices could provide the impetus to replace physicians in certain specialties, such as radiology and pathology, with a "new breed" of data science–savvy specialists who would embrace and harness AI's potential.

- Affecting the fundamental values of empathy, compassion, and trust in a patient-centered, relational healthcare model: The ability of AI to improve healthcare efficiency and accuracy could potentially allow physicians more time to provide care with greater empathy, compassion, and trust.

SUMMARY

This chapter delineates the concept of AI as an introduction to the two subsequent chapters dealing with the applications of AI in cutaneous imaging and histopathology. The term "AI" was thoroughly defined, followed by depiction of the history of AI, commercial investment in AI, and some detailed and non-technical discussions on the principles of two common AI methods utilized in medicine: machine learning and deep learning (neural network). To conclude the chapter, ethical considerations and potential unintended consequences of AI application in medicine were discussed.

REFERENCES

1. [MERRIAM-WEBSTER]. Definition of intelligence. Merriam-Webster Dictionary. 2020a. [www.merriam-webster.com/dictionary/intelligence] Accessed May 11, 2020.
2. [CAMBRIDGE]. Intelligence. Cambridge Dictionary. 2020a. [https://dictionary.cambridge.org/us/dictionary/English/intelligence] Accessed May 11, 2020.
3. [CAMBRIDGE]. Intelligence. Cambridge Dictionary. 2020b. [https://dictionary.cambridge.org/us/dictionary/English/artificial] Accessed May 11, 2020.
4. [MERRIAM-WEBSTER]. Definition of intelligence. Merriam-Webster Dictionary. 2020b. [www.merriam-webster.com/dictionary/artificial] Accessed May 11, 2020.
5. Ertel W. *Introduction to Artificial Intelligence*. 2nd Ed. Springer, Cham, Switzerland, 2017.
6. Kerasidou A. Artificial intelligence and the ongoing need for empathy, compassion and trust in healthcare. *Bull World Health Organ* 2020; 98(4): 245–250. Doi: 10.2471/BLT.19.237198.
7. Wilson HJ and Daugherty PR. Collaborative intelligence: Humans and AI are joining forces. *Harvard Business Review* 2018; July–August.
8. [COMPUTER HISTORY MUSEUM]. The 1956 Dartmouth workshop and its immediate consequences: The origins of artificial intelligence. Computer History Museum. [www.computerhistory.org/events/1956-dartmouth-workshop-its-immediate/] Accessed May 14, 2020.

9. McCarthy J, Abrahams PW, Edwards DJ, et al. *LISP 1.5 program manual*. MIT Press, Cambridge, MA, 1962.
10. Knight W. *What Marvin Minsky Still Means for AI*. MIT Technology Review, Cambridge, MA, January 26, 2016.
11. Samuel AL. Some studies in machine learning using the game of checkers. *IBM J Res Develop* 1959; 3(3): 210–229. Doi: 10.1147/rd.33.0210.
12. Award M and Khanna R. *Efficient Learning Machines*. Apress (Open Access), Berkeley, CA, 2015.
13. Myers A. Stanford's John McCarthy, seminal figure of artificial intelligence, dies at 84. *Stanford News*. October 25, 2011. [https://news.stanford.edu/news/2011/October/john-mccarthy-obit-102511.html] Accessed May 15, 2020.
14. Haykin S. *Neural Networks*. Prentice Hall, Upper Saddle River, NJ, 1994.
15. Yao X. Evolving artificial neural networks. *Proc IEEE* 1999; 87: 1423–1447.
16. LeCun Y, Bengio Y, and Hinton G. Deep learning. *Nature* 2015; 521: 436–444.
17. Bera K, Schalper KA, Rimm DL, et al. Artificial intelligence in digital pathology—new tools for diagnosis and precision oncology. *Nat Rev Clin Oncol* 2019; 16(11): 703–715. Doi: 10.1038/s41571-019-0252-y.
18. [MIT NEWS] IBM and MIT to pursue joint research in artificial intelligence, establish new MIT-IBM Watson AI Lab. September 7, 2017. [news.mit.edu/2017/ibm-mit-joint-research-watson-artificial-intelligence-lab-0907]   Accessed June 2, 2020.
19. Dizikes P. Institute launches the MIT intelligence quest: New institute-wide initiative will advance human and machine intelligence research. *MIT News*. February 1, 2018. [news.mit.edu/mit-launches-intelligence-quest-0201] Accessed June 2, 2020.
20. Amoroso A. In focus: How AI is reshaping the future—and our investments. September 26, 2019. J.P. Morgan Private Bank. [privatebank.jpmorgan.com] Accessed June 17, 2020.
21. Reif LR. Transformative automation is coming. The impact is up to us. *Boston Globe*. November 10, 2017. [www.bostonglobe.com/opinion/2017/11/10/transformative-automation-coming-the-impact/az0qppTvsUu5VUKJyQvoSN/story.html] Accessed July 5, 2020.
22. Michalski RS. A theory and methodology of inductive learning. *Artificial Intelligence* 1983; 20: 111–118.
23. Kearns M and Roth A. *The Ethical Algorithm: The Science of Socially Aware Algorithm Design*. Oxford University Press, Oxford, 2020.
24. Fine TL. Book review: Fundamentals of artificial neural networks—M.H. Hassoun (Cambridge, MA: MIT Press, 1995). *IEEE. Transactions on Information Theory* 1996; 42(4): 1322–1324.
25. Agatonovic-Kustrin S and Beresford R. Basic concepts of artificial neural network (ANN) modeling and its application in pharmaceutical research. *Biomedical Analysis* 2000; 22(5): 717–727.
26. Trafton A. Artificial intelligence yields new antibiotics: A deep-learning model identifies a powerful new drug that can kill many species of antibiotic-resistant bacteria. *MIT News* 2020; February 20.
27. Benke K and Benke G. Artificial intelligence and big data in public health. *Int J Environ Res Public Health* 2018; 15(12): 2796. Doi: 10.3390/ijerph15122796.

28. Hueso M, Vellido A, Montero N, et al. Artificial intelligence for the artificial kidney: Pointers to the future of a personalized hemodialysis therapy. *Kidney Dis (Basel)* 2018; 4(1): 1–9. Doi: 10.1159/0000486394.

29. Panch T, Szolovits P, and Atun R. Artificial intelligence, machine learning and health systems. *J Glob Health* 2018; 8(2): 020303. Doi: 10.7189/jogh.08.020303.

30. Mirchi N, Bissonnette V, Yilmaz R, et al. The virtual operative assistant: An explainable artificial intelligence tool for simulation-based training in surgery and medicine. *PLoS One* 2020; 15(2): e0229596. Doi: 10.1371/journal.pone. 0229596.

31. Topol E. *Deep Medicine: How Artificial Intelligence Can Make Healthcare Human Again.* Basic Books, New York, 2019.

32. Pasquale F. *The Black Box Society: The Secret Algorithms That Control Money and Information.* Harvard University Press, Cambridge, MA, 2015.

33. O'Neil C. *Weapons of Math Destruction: How Big Data Increases Inequality and Threatens Democracy.* Broadway Books, New York, 2017.

34. Snow J. Bias already exists in search engine results, and it's only going to get worse. *MIT Tech Review.* February 26, 2018.

35. Noble S. *Algorithms of Oppression: How Search Engines Reinforce Racism.* 1st Ed. New York University Press, New York, 2018.

36. Zuboff S. *The Age of Surveillance Capitalism: The Fight for a Human Future at the New Frontier of Power.* PublicAffairs, New York, 2020.

37. Baroe K, Miyata-Sturm A, and Handen E. How to achieve trustworthy artificial intelligence for health. *Bull World Health Organ* 2020; 98(4): 257–262. Doi: 10.2471/BLT.19.237289.

38. Cabitza F, Rasoini R, and Gensini GF. Unintended consequences of machine learning in medicine. *JAMA* 2017; 318: 517–518.

39. Chan S and Siegel EL. Will machine learning end the viability of radiology as a thriving medical specialty? *Br J Radiol* 2019; 92(1094): 20180416. Doi: 10.11259/bjr.20180416.

Artificial Intelligence in Cutaneous Imaging

Lawrence S. Chan

Contents

DOI: 10.1201/9781003121275-3

INTRODUCTION

This chapter deals with the subject of utilizing artificial intelligence (AI) for cutaneous imaging. Unlike most medical specialties, imaging is essentially the "heart and soul" of the specialty of dermatology. What you see is what you get, so to speak. Our specialty places a huge emphasis on visual inspection as a critical diagnostic component, right from the start of professional training. When I served as a dermatology resident at the University of Michigan Medical Center, the first-year resident physicians were assigned to silently examine patients, wrote down the findings of our visual inspection, and then presented those observations to the faculty members to discuss the diagnosis at the weekly clinical grand rounds, a typical clinical didactic teaching session [1]. Conversation with patients during grand rounds was prohibited. As a result of such strong emphasis on visual examination, the trained residents commonly developed a keen observational skill that will last the lifetime of their dermatology practice. Some of those skills we learned, include skin lesions' individual shape, group configuration, color, size, surface change, and location, were especially important for our professional daily care of patients, as they helped us narrow down the diagnostic possibilities. After we finished our residency training, we took the qualifying examination administered by the American Board of Dermatology for professional certification. Again, the examination tested our visual inspection skills through questions based on images of skin lesions, which comprise nearly 50% of the examination contents. Along with a passing score on general knowledge of dermatology and a passing score on histopathology of skin diseases, a passing score on visual images of dermatology secured a board certification for the graduated dermatology residents. Image is, indeed, critical to the dermatology specialty.

ANALYSIS OF THE NEED

Having stated the importance of visual examination in the profession of dermatology, we now turn to the question of whether there is a need to involve AI to help us making visual diagnoses of skin diseases. As the computer scientist Elaine Rich stated, "Artificial intelligence is the study of how to make computers do things at which, at the moment, people are better" [2]; this is exactly what we will be focusing on. Accordingly, this chapter is not about asking AI to help us perform something we skin physicians cannot do, but rather to improve our performance. In this case, it is about the possibility of an improvement in diagnostic accuracy for skin diseases and an enhancement of healthcare delivery.

One clear advantage of AI-assisted skin imaging is its ability to conduct telemedicine practice. Dermatology services in rural America are in short supply. It was estimated that only 10% of dermatologists practice in rural America in a study published in 2018 [3]. And the trend of dermatologists' practice geography is not encouraging either. A paper published in 2018 revealed that dermatologist density increased by 21% from 1995 (3.02 per 100,000 population) to 2013 (3.65 per 100,000 population) nationwide. This seemingly good news did not improve the access to dermatology care in rural America. While dermatologist density (provider per 100,000 population) increased substantially from 3.47 to 4.11 in urban areas, it only increased minimally, from 0.065 to 0.085, in rural areas. Consequently, the provider density gap between urban and rural areas actually increased from 3.41 (per 100,000) to 4.03 (per 100,000) during this time period, indicating an increasing tendency of dermatologists to locate their practices in urban communities over rural areas [4]. Thus, this workforce disparity, important for rural patient care in dermatology, is actually getting worse over time. The application of AI-assisted diagnosis method on digital cutaneous images, which can be taken in rural location and forwarded to distant centers for disease determination, may have a role in narrowing this service gap. In this regard, AI-assisted skin cancer screening may serve as a good triage tool that can help filter out benign lesions, thus allowing more efficient management of cancerous lesions. In doing so, the access to dermatology care in rural America would be improved [5].

Another possible advantage of AI-assisted skin imaging is its potential to improve skin cancer diagnostics. A recent paper reported that the AI method can achieve a diagnostic accuracy that is on par with fully trained and American Board of Dermatology–certified dermatologists [6]. If we consider that the AI-assisted method, trained with bigger databases and appropriate algorithm adjustment, might continue to get better and become more accurate over time and that fully trained board-certified dermatologists are already at the peak of their diagnostic ability, the AI-assisted method could potentially perform a better job on this kind of cancer diagnosis, being more accurate and even more efficient.

Considering all skin cancers, the deadliest one is melanoma. However, it is easily curable if the diagnosis and treatment are performed at an early disease stage. According to a paper published in 2014, the incidence of melanoma continues to increase worldwide, and this trend poses great healthcare and socio-economical problems [7]. In fact, the incidence of melanoma is increasing at a rate faster than any other form of skin cancer and it accounts for the majority of skin cancer–related deaths [8, 9]. The average lifetime risk for melanoma has reached 1 in 50 in many Western countries [10]. When melanoma is detected early, such as in stage 1, patients have a 95% five-year survival rate, which quickly drops to a rate ranging from 8% to 20% if the cancer reaches the higher disease stages [9]. Since delaying diagnosis and the corresponding timely treatment will likely result in metastasis, treatment complications, and high mortality, the key for melanoma management is to make early detection and perform appropriate surgical treatment accordingly. At the present time, physicians make clinical diagnosis of melanoma predominantly based on visual recognition of abnormal pigmented patterns present in melanoma that set it apart from benign melanocytic nevus. However, the clear black-and-white characteristics distinguishing melanoma from nevus by visual inspection are not always present, as clinical lesions exhibit a various spectrum of "gray" shape features that can be observed in both benign lesions and cancerous ones. This diagnostic difficulty encountered by physicians is revealed by the stunningly low percentages (3%–25%, mean 10%) of clinically suspected melanoma being confirmed at the histopathological level. With the aid of a dermoscope (a handheld microscope), physicians well trained in the use of this device can pick up melanoma with a sensitivity as high as 98%, but with a low specificity of 68%, in some studies [11]. Therefore, the current method of diagnosis is still not optimal for detecting early melanoma in a highly sensitive and specific manner. The available AI-assisted diagnosis methods prompt us to examine whether such novel methods will improve physicians' ability to pick up early melanoma lesions while sparing the benign ones. We will examine recently published studies outlining these AI-assisted skin cancer diagnostics, particularly for melanoma. We will be focusing on the applications of two commonly utilized AI algorithms: machine learning (ML) and deep learning (DL).

THE TECHNOLOGY: AI APPLICATIONS IN CUTANEOUS IMAGING

ML for Melanoma Screening

In 2016, researchers published an examination of the validity of using ML to generate a quantitative image analysis [11]. They asked the following questions:

- What are the sensitivity and specificity of the automated image analysis?
- Can the melanoma imaging biomarkers (MIBs) generated by automated imaging analysis of pigmented lesions exhibit spectral dependence for improving diagnosis?

Accordingly, they set up the following experimental designs:

- 120 images of dermoscopic examination were utilized for this study, consisting of 60 melanomas and 60 atypical nevi.
- These images were analyzed by a series of computerized programs, measuring the lesions' border, center, and a 360-degree sweep from the center. By plotting the image's brightness versus a 45-degree sweep and using blue channel color information, graphic data was generated for MIB use.
- Other computerized programs determine lesional symmetry, pigment pattern organization, networks, and substructures across tricolor channels: red, green, and blue.
- Additional programs measure the number of different colors present and the pattern of the pigment network.
- Together, these computerized programs run on each image generate 50 quantitative metrics. Thirty-three of these 50 metrics, found to have statistically significant difference in value between melanomas and nevi, were selected to be the MIB set.
- Assayed through particular color channels, MIBs then became the basic data for the analysis by a set of 13 ML classification algorithms to construct overall quantitative scores (Q-scores), ranging from zero (least likely to be melanoma) to one (most likely to be melanoma).

Their study results revealed the following:

- Most skin lesions with high Q-scores were correctly determined to be melanomas, and most lesions with low Q-scores were accurately diagnosed as benign nevi.
- This classification method has achieved 98% sensitivity and 36% specificity in making a correct diagnosis of melanoma.

Therefore, they concluded that this AI-driven method has the potential to improve our melanoma diagnostic capability and that more adjustment of the AI application is needed.

Deep Neural Networks for Skin Cancer Classification

Using a deep convolutional neural network (CNN) type of AI (a deep learning (DL) AI), another group of researchers demonstrated that AI could achieve skin cancer classification at board-certified dermatologists' level of competence [6]. The following are the study methods:

- These researchers utilized a single CNN to train the computer with an end-to-end method using images (clinical and dermoscopic) directly.
- The rationale for utilizing a CNN type of AI is that CNN has the potential to distinguish lesions across many fine-grained object categories, a challenging task when using automation for classifying skin lesions with substantial fine-grained variability.
- Images were collected from 18 different open-access physician-curated online repositories and clinical data from Stanford University Medical Center. The dataset contains 2,032 different physician-labeled diseases in 757 disease classes.
- The entire dataset was separated into two subsets: 127,463 clinical images for training and validation, and 1,942 clinical images (biopsy labeled) for testing. The dataset also included 3,374 dermoscopic images.
- The inputs for the AI were raw pixels and disease labels.
- After training the AI CNN, the researchers then tested the ability of the CNN, in comparison to 21 board-certified dermatologists, on biopsy-proven clinical images of two binary and critical use cases: a case of keratinocyte-origin carcinoma against seborrheic keratosis and a case of malignant melanoma against melanocytic nevi. In addition, the test was also performed for classification of melanoma on dermoscopic images.

Their studies yielded the following results:

- Overall, the performance of the CNN matched or exceeded that of 21 dermatologists tested on three critical diagnostic tasks: distinguishing keratinocyte carcinoma from benign keratosis on a clinical image, classifying melanoma from benign nevus on a clinical image, and determining melanoma from benign nevus by a dermoscopic image.

Therefore, this study clearly illustrates a great potential for AI in assisting skin cancer diagnosis.

Another Diagnostic Battle of Man against Machine

This study pits AI, a DL type of convolutional neural network (CNN), against 58 dermatologists in a melanoma diagnosis challenge [5, 12]. The methods of the study were:

- A test set of 300 dermoscopic images was generated.
- The set included melanomas of both in-situ and invasive types in all body sites, comprising 20% of the set.
- The remaining (80%) component of set contained benign nevi of various types in different body sites. Approximately 75% of this component was judged to be benign based on a follow-up monitor but not documented by histology.
- Training samples for CNN were separated from samples used for validation.
- 100 images were selected by two experts from the 300-image set for testing purposes.
- 172 dermatologists from the International Dermoscopy Society were invited to participate, and 58 of the invitees submitted answers.
- For level-I evaluation, participants were provided only with 100 dermoscopic images and were asked to provide diagnosis of either melanoma or nevus.
- For level-II evaluation, which occurred four weeks post-level-I evaluation, participants were provided with the same 100 dermoscopic images plus close-up images of same and additional clinical information.
- Statistical analysis was conducted to measure receiver operating characteristic (ROC) area under the curve (AUC), as well as sensitivity and specificity. Statistical significance was also determined.

The results of the study indicated that:

- The CNN achieved a ROC AUC of 0.86, which was higher than the mean ROC AUC achieved by dermatologists (0.79, $p < 0.01$).
- At sensitivity level of 86.6%, the CNN achieved a higher specificity than that of the dermatologists for level-I evaluation (82.5% vs. 71.3%, $p < 0.01$).

- At sensitivity level of 88.9%, the CNN similarly achieved a higher specificity than that of the dermatologists for level-II evaluation (82.5% vs. 75.7%, $p < 0.01$).

Thus, this study concludes that CNN could outperform most dermatologists in diagnosing melanoma on dermoscopic images. And CNN did it at a statistically significant level.

More Studies Documenting CNN Outperforming Dermatologists

In a paper published in 2019, a DL type of AI CNN was shown to outperform 112 dermatologists in melanoma diagnosis [13]. Aiming to reflect the real-life clinical experience in which multiple diagnoses are considered when encountering patients, this study utilized the following methods:

- 11,444 dermoscopic images were initially collected, comprising the major pigmented skin lesions taken by different camera systems of heterogeneous patient populations, both benign and malignant, and were used to prepare the training set. Duplications were screened and removed from the image set. The number of biopsy-proven images in the set was 6,390. This AI training set included diseases in five major categories: 1) melanocytic nevi, 2) melanoma, 3) basal cell carcinoma, 4) benign keratoses (seborrheic keratosis, solar lentigo, lichenoid keratosis), and 5) squamous cell lesions (actinic keratosis, Bowen disease, squamous cell carcinoma). The final training set of 12,336 images consisted of 4,219; 3,521; 910; 3,101; and 585 images of the diseases in the above designated categories 1, 2, 3, 4, and 5, respectively.
- A set of 300 dermoscopic images, which were proven by histology, was utilized to test the performance of CNN against that of 112 dermatologists (median four years' practice in dermatology) from 13 different German university hospitals. This set is composed of 60 cases for each of the five categories of disease mentioned earlier. Each image is evaluated by at least 14 dermatologists, and up to 30.
- The primary end-point was the determination of a correct diagnosis between benign nevi and melanoma, with a secondary end-point being correct classification of one of the five diagnostic categories mentioned earlier.

The outcomes of this study revealed that:

- For the primary end-point results: Dermatologists achieved an overall sensitivity of 74.4% (95% confidence interval at 67.0–81.8%) and a specificity of 59.8% (95% confidence interval at 49.8–69.8%). At the same sensitivity level of 74.4%, CNN outperformed dermatologists for a specificity of 91.3% (95% confidence interval at 85.5–97.1%). Two-side McNemar tests confirmed a statistical significance (p < 0.001).
- For the secondary end-point data: Dermatologists obtained an overall sensitivity of 56.5% (95% confidence interval at 42.8–70.2%) and a specificity of 89.2% (95% confidence interval at 85.0–93.3%). At the identical sensitivity level of 56.5%, CNN similarly outperformed dermatologists for a specificity of 98.8%. This difference was statistically significant by two-side McNemar test (p < 0.001), with the exception of basal cell carcinoma determination (an on-par performance).

Thus, more studies point to the possibility that AI can assist dermatologists in achieving a clinically meaningful determination of pigmented and non-pigmented skin lesions when encountering multiple classes of skin diseases.

More Neural Networks for Identification of Melanoma on Dermoscopic Images

In a study published in 2020, researchers examined the abilities of an AI neural network called DERM (deep ensemble for recognition of melanoma, a DL type of AI) to detect melanoma in human pigmented lesion collections [9]. Their objective was to assess the accuracy of AI in identifying melanoma from dermoscopic images and to compare the physicians' performance with that of AI by meta-analysis. The methods of their studies were as follows:

- DERM was created and developed specifically for identification of pigmentary features associated with melanoma.
- The deep learning method of DERM directly "learned" from original data, rather than using predetermined features.
- The image datasets found to contain bias and images determined to be identical or near-identical were excluded. The final inclusion of 7,120 dermoscopic images of the gold-standard pathologically

validated melanoma (24%) and benign pigmented lesions (76%) were used to train and test the AI system.

- The DERM algorithm was trained and validated against the datasets using a "10-fold cross-validation" method, which ensured that every image was examined once and that the same image is not used for both training and testing.
- The cross-validation was carried out by dividing the datasets into several "folds," with each fold used to tested the algorithm. The results collected from each fold were then averaged.
- The AI DERM program generated a numerical response score ranging from 0 (meaning near zero confidence of being melanoma) to 1 (meaning near 100% confidence of being melanoma). A non-parametric receiver operating characteristics (ROC) area under the curve (AUC) was used to test the overall accuracy, using histopathology as gold standard.
- Unlike other studies that compare the AI method with a limited panel of physicians on the same datasets, meta-analysis was conducted to compare the accuracy of diagnosis by DERM with that of dermatologists and general physicians, with or without the aid of a handheld dermoscope.

The results of their studies showed the following:

- The AI DERM program achieved a maximum AUC of 0.93 (95% confidence interval at 0.922–0.928), with 85% sensitivity and 85% specificity. To avoid false negativity in making the all-important melanoma determination, the AI DERM can achieve a 95% sensitivity with a reduced specificity of 64% or a 99% sensitivity with a low specificity of 47%.
- The DERM program performance was nearly identical to human experts' (dermatologists') performance with the aid of dermoscopy (maximum AUC of 0.91, sensitivity 85%, specificity 85%) and was slightly better than experts' performance without dermoscopy (maximum AUC of 0.90, sensitivity 79%, specificity 86%). As expected, experts' performances were better than those of non-experts.

Like the results reported in the *Nature* paper [6], this study confirmed that AI, particularly the DL type, can achieve a high performance on par with that of dermatologists.

UNFINISHED BUSINESS

For the AI-assisted method to become a viable day-to-day melanoma diagnosis technique, the society needs to resolve several important issues: patients' trust of this method, medical-legal issues, and proper health insurance coverage.

Patients' Trust

Regardless how good the AI-assisted method can become in the future, it cannot be accepted as a viable clinical tool without the patients' trust. The patients' trust, in turn, depends on solid clinical data support. Such supportive clinical data would also increase the confidence of physicians, who will be in the interface between patients they care for and the AI applications.

Medical-Legal Considerations

Second, the medical-legal issues in utilizing the AI-assisted method also need a resolution [14, 15]. In the unlikely scenario of diagnostic error while utilizing AI method, which party would bear the ultimate responsibility: the physician, the computer maker, or the AI programmer? This issue needs to be settled before the AI method can go "mainstream" for skin cancer diagnosis. This is especially critical for melanoma, the misdiagnosis of which could result in high chance of mortality.

Health Insurance Coverage

In addition to resolving the trust and legal issues, physicians need proper health insurance coverage for this AI-assisted method. There could possibly be some added expense in applying the AI-assisted method. Would insurance agencies compensate physicians for their additional costs for the new technology?

SUMMARY

Analysis of the few available published articles on the use of AI for clinical dermatology has allowed us to perform a preliminary assessment of AI's

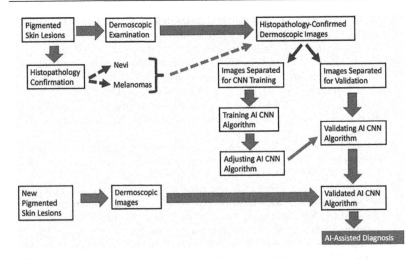

FIGURE 2.1 A schematic flow of a potential AI-assisted melanoma diagnostic approach. (CNN = convolutional neural network.)

ability in this aspect of medicine. Thus far, the DL type of AI applications, such as CNN, appear to be better at this task than the ML type of AI. Most of these studies, however, were based on images taken by dermoscope, and not clinical images taken by simple photography. Although dermoscopic images provide a level of standardization, obtaining such images adds another layer of complexity. The results of these studies thus far provide evidence that AI could perform on par with dermatologists or even superior to dermatologists in making diagnoses of malignant melanoma. As we anticipate further improvement of AI in clinical dermatology diagnosis, we also need to consider other related issues of patients' trust, medical-legal consideration, and insurance coverage before the AI-assisted method can become a "standard of care." See Figure 2.1.

REFERENCES

1. [DIDACTICS]. Didactics. Residency program. Dermatology. Michigan Medicine. [https://medicine.umich.edu/dept/dermatology/education/residency-program/didactics] Accessed May 17, 2020.
2. Rich E. *Artificial Intelligence.* McGraw-Hill, New York, 1983.

3. Vaidya T, Zubritsky L, Alikhan A, and Housholder A. Socioeconomic and geographic barriers to dermatology care in urban and rural US populations. *J Am Acad Dermatol* 2018; 78(2): 406–408. Doi: 10.1016/j.jaad.2017.07.050.

4. Feng H, Berk-Krauss J, Feng PW, and Stein JA. Comparison of dermatologist density between urban and rural counties in the United States. *JAMA Dermatol* 2018; 154(11): 1265–1271. Doi: 10.1001/jamadermatol.2018.3022.

5. Mar VJ and Soyer HP. Artificial intelligence for melanoma diagnosis: How can we deliver on the promise? *Ann Oncol* 2018; 29(8): 1625–1628. Doi: 10.1093/annonc/mdy193.

6. Esteva A, Kuprel B, Novoa RA, Ko J, Swetter SM, Blau HM, and Thrun S. Dermatologist-level classification of skin cancer with deep neural networks. *Nature* 2017; 542(7639): 115–118. Doi: 10.1038/nature21056.

7. Rastrelli M, Tropea S, Rossi CR, and Alaibac M. Melanoma: Epidemiology, risk factors, pathogenesis and classification. *In Vivo* 2014; 28(6): 1005–1011.

8. Marsden JR, Newton-Bishop JA, Burrows L, et al. Revised UK guidelines for the management of cutaneous melanoma. *Br J Dermatol* 2010; 163(2): 238–256.

9. Phillips M, Greenhalgh J, Marsden H, et al. Detection of malignant melanoma using artificial intelligence: An observational study of diagnostic accuracy. *Dermatol Pract Concept* 2020; 10(1): e2020011. Doi: 10.5826/dpc.1001a11.

10. Meyle KD and Guldberg P. Genetic risk factors for melanoma. *Hum Genet* 2009; 4: 499–510.

11. Gareau DS, da Rosa JC, Yagerman S, et al. Digital imaging biomarkers feed machine learning for melanoma screening. *Exp Dermatol* 2016; 26(7). https://doi.org/10.1111/exd.13250.

12. Haenssle HA, Fink C, Schneiderbauer R, et al. Man against machine: Diagnostic performance of a deep learning convolutional neural network for dermoscopic melanoma recognition in comparison to 58 dermatologists. *Ann Oncol* 2018; 29(8): 1836–1842.

13. Maron RC, Weichenthal M, Utikal JS, et al. Systematic outperformance of 112 dermatologists in multiclass skin cancer image classification by convolutional neural networks. *Eur J Cancer* 2019; 119: 57–65. https://doi.org/10.1016/ejca.2019.06.013.

14. Goldberg DJ. Legal issues in dermatology: Informed consent, complications and medical malpractice. *Semin Cutan Med Surg* 2007; 26(1): 2–5. Doi: 10.1016/j.sder.2006.12.001.

15. Carter SM, Rogers W, Win KT, et al. The ethical, legal and social implications of using artificial intelligence system in breast cancer care. *The Breast* 2020; 49: 25–32. https://doi.10.1016/j.breast.2019.10.001.

Artificial Intelligence in Cutaneous Histopathology

Lawrence S. Chan

Contents

DOI: 10.1201/9781003121275-4

INTRODUCTION

Pathology is a medical specialty that studies the nature and makes diagnoses of diseases. The term "pathology" is a word derived from two Greek-language roots: *pathos*, meaning suffering or disease, and *logia*, meaning communication, writing, or subject of study [1]. The large field of pathology is commonly divided into three major branches based on functionality: 1) clinical pathology, 2) anatomic pathology, and 3) molecular pathology. While clinical pathology services perform studies to examine disease manifestations in bodily fluid (blood, urine, wound and central nervous system fluid), anatomic pathology studies and makes diagnosis of diseases in tissue, in organs, and sometimes in whole body levels. Molecular pathology, a recently developed branch, determines disease at the molecular level by utilizing advanced molecular biological techniques (such as in-situ hybridization and polymerase chain reaction). This chapter focuses on one specific area of anatomic pathology: histopathology. Histopathology is a pathology discipline that deals with anatomic structure affected by disease at the tissue level. It has long been considered the gold standard for diagnosis of disease at the tissue level, when a definite diagnosis cannot be made by clinical inspection alone [2]. Pathologists are considered, appropriately, to be "doctors' doctors" [3].

The use of histopathology for examination of skin disease started around the 1940s. One of the pioneers of cutaneous histopathology was a German-born, American-educated physician named Walter F. Lever, who is commonly referred as the founder of cutaneous pathology. Dr. Lever, who was trained both in cutaneous pathology and biochemistry, authored the very first textbook on skin pathology, with the earliest edition published in 1949 [4]. The many important pathology contributions Dr. Lever offered to the field of dermatology include distinguishing pemphigus (a life-threatening, intra-epidermal blistering disease) from bullous pemphigoid (a non-life-threatening, sub-epidermal blistering disease); ultrastructural and biochemical characterizations of appendage tumors of the skin; ultrastructural depiction of acantholysis (epidermal cell separation in pemphigus group of diseases); and ultrastructural delineation of antibody-binding location in autoimmune blistering diseases [5]. Since that time, cutaneous pathology has become an important and integral part of dermatology training and practice. In fact, graduating dermatology resident physicians will need to pass the histopathology part of the examination, as well as clinical part of the test, in order to receive certification of competence from the American Board of

Dermatology, the most reputable certifying agency for dermatology professionals in the United States [6].

The basic cutaneous pathology method is to prepare skin samples, which are preserved in formalin. The samples are hardened in paraffin (a wax-like compound); sliced into thin sections; placed onto glass slides; and stained with a mixture of a chemical stain compound called hematoxylin/eosin, which renders cell nuclei dark blue and most cell cytoplasm light red. The dermatopathologist—the histopathologist specializing in skin diseases—then examines those stained sections under a conventional light microscope to determine the diagnosis. Additional pathology techniques used in the diagnosis of cutaneous diseases include special staining with paraffinized sections, electron microscopy, immunohistochemistry, and immunofluorescence microscopy. Special stains are utilized to delineate critical diagnostic components not identified by hematoxylin/eosin stain, such as fungi (by Grocott (methanmine) silver stain), mycobacteria (by Ziehl-Neelsen stain), mucin (by Alcian blue stain), and amyloid (by Congo red stain). Electron microscopy is used to examine the ultrastructure of the skin and its components, whereas the immunohistochemistry method is used to detect certain components or cell types by antibody, and immunofluorescence microscopy is utilized to determine the immune nature of the diseases. More recently, newer and more advanced molecular methods, such as polymerase chain reaction and flowcytometry, have been incorporated with traditional pathology techniques for determining certain disease conditions [7]. Nowadays, cutaneous pathology is essential for dermatology specialty because of the following functions it performs:

- Guides physicians to an accurate diagnosis
- Confirms or rules out skin cancer
- Evaluates the depth and the invasion of skin cancer in the disease-stage determination
- Substantiates or discards a cutaneous metastasis of internal malignancy
- Determines or rejects a life-threatening blistering disorder
- Defines separating location of a blistering disease at the ultrastructural level
- Distinguishes types of blistering diseases
- Establishes or dismisses a dangerous drug eruption
- Endorses or discounts a cutaneous manifestation of systemic disease
- Verifies or disproves an infectious disease
- Authenticates or invalidates a medical-legal challenge

The importance of cutaneous histopathology is such that correct diagnosis of many skin diseases depends on it. At times, the life of a patient rests on a correct pathology diagnosis made in a timely manner. Melanoma, a skin cancer carrying a high mortality rate, and toxic epidermal necrolysis, a life-threatening skin reaction resembling a burn condition, are two such examples.

ANALYSIS OF THE NEED

Having stated the essential function of cutaneous histopathology in the practice of dermatology and care of patients with skin diseases, our next question is why the need for AI-assisted cutaneous histopathology? Just as we discussed in the last chapter about AI-assisted clinical imaging, our focus on this chapter is not so much about asking AI to assist us to achieve something we physicians cannot perform at the present time, but rather inquiring if AI can help improving our diagnosis accuracy and efficiency from the perspective of histopathology diagnostics and healthcare delivery.

Drawbacks of Our Current State of Histopathology

The Subjectivity of Threshold

The substantial contribution of cutaneous histopathology to the field of dermatology notwithstanding, there are some drawbacks. First, skin histopathology, like histopathology of other tissue types, is based on "threshold" findings for diagnostic determination. That means that a pathology specimen is judged on whether the microscopic observations have reached a certain criterion "threshold" to be considered for certain diagnosis. This diagnostic "threshold," in turn, is heavily influenced by the training a given pathologist received from his or her mentor. Since different mentors may have trained their mentees with "thresholds" that are slightly different, this leads to an inherent subjectivity, resulting in variability of diagnostic determination across the spectrum of practice [2]. In addition, the natural differences in visual perception, data integration, and judgement between independent pathologists would inevitably lead to discrepancy in opinion; inconsistency in diagnosis; and, ultimately, suboptimal patient care. A Canadian author humorously described pathology this way: "Under the pathologist's microscope, life and death fight in an illuminated circle in a sort of cellular bullfight. The pathologist's job is to find the bull among the matador cells" [8]. In short, there is no absolute standard. The AI-assisted pathology approach, which is more robust and reproducible, could be a starting point to remedy the challenges of variability and inconsistency we face in our current state of cutaneous histopathology [9]. This subjectivity problem will remain even with the implementation of digital pathology, which is detailed in the paragraphs that follow.

The Impediment of Information Transfer Speed

When a dermatopathologist encounters a difficult case and is not confident in rendering a final diagnosis, the next step he or she would logically consider is to send the case to a consultant for a second opinion. The conventional process requires the stained glass slides to be transported physically from one location to another: from the pathology laboratory to the pathologist's office, from one pathologist's office to a consulting pathologist's office, and so on. Thus, the diagnosis process may be delayed for days or weeks [4]. The availability of digital pathology will help solve this speed problem.

Advantage of AI-Assisted Pathology for Enabling Telemedicine

Just as dermatologists are in short supply in the American rural areas, dermatopathologists rarely practice in rural communities [2]. Digital pathology may help bridge the service gap in those needed areas through the telemedicine approach. A sequence of events like the following can be helpful and practical. A skin biopsy performed in a rural setting can be processed locally; the hemotaxylin/eosin-stained tissue sections on glass slides can be scanned into digital images, which can then be sent via the internet to an urban cutaneous histopathology center for determination; and the diagnosis made is e-transmitted back to the rural physician. AI-assisted cutaneous pathology, along with digital pathology, will provide an even better way, in a manner of semi-automation, to serve the rural communities as we will discuss in the paragraphs that follow.

THE TECHNOLOGY: AI-ASSISTED CUTANEOUS HISTOPATHOLOGY

Having discussed the importance of histopathology in dermatology and the possible usefulness of AI-assisted cutaneous histopathology, we will now describe some usages of AI in histopathology. Since 2015, many publications have documented the use of AI for pathology [9–18]. Although a focused study of AI application in cutaneous histopathology has not been depicted in the Pubmed-based literature, the applicability of AI in histopathology of other tissue types should be easily transferrable to cutaneous histopathology.

General Principles of Digital Histopathology

Before discussing AI-assisted histopathology, a brief description of digital pathology, the basic element that enables AI-assisted histopathology, would be helpful. Since the first digital camera prototype was developed by an engineer at Eastman Kodak in 1975, it has now become the dominant photographic image equipment, with the near disappearance of all new film camera production [19]. It is therefore not surprising that histopathology, a medical sub-field that is totally image based, is also being dominated by digital applications. In fact, a professional organization, the Digital Pathology Association, was established in 2009 to serve the professional needs of over 1,000 members, including pathologists, scientists, technologists, and pathology-related industry representatives. According to the website of this association, digital pathology is defined as "a dynamic, image-based environment that enables the acquisition, management and interpretation of pathology information generated from a digitalized glass slide" [20]. Typically, digital pathology employs a whole slide scanner (a digital microscope) outfitted with a high-resolution camera and special software and optical equipment. The scanning of the stained tissue on a glass slide produces a digital image file called whole slide imaging (WSI). Since the quality of these WSIs is critical for diagnostic purposes, the US Food and Drug Administration has participated in the approval process of commercial scanners, providing assurance of the image quality [3, 21]. In fact, several studies have confirmed that diagnoses made utilizing digital images revealed little or no difference from those rendered by conventional microscopic examination [3, 22, 23]. This digitalized image can then be sent to pathologists for diagnostic viewing. The easy transport of a digital image through the internet therefore facilitates the diagnostic process, especially when additional histopathology consultants in a far-distant location are needed for difficult cases or sought for a second diagnostic opinion. The recent maturity of digital pathology therefore paves a timely pathway for the current development of AI-assisted histopathology [3].

Specific Applications of AI-Assisted Histopathology

The next step in utilizing digital pathology is to enlist AI to facilitate diagnostic decision support by increasing the workflow speed and accuracy of the diagnostic process. Some published reports on AI applications for histopathological diagnosis that produce positive results are discussed next.

As early as 2011, researchers have combined AI with pathology in an attempt to achieve a predictive model for breast cancer prognosis, even with conventional glass slides for AI training purposes [3, 24]. Targeting a set of quantifiable features within breast cancer histology, the researchers generated a computer algorithm to train with the data, which were then used to create a prognostic prediction model. Utilizing this model, the researchers analyzed 676 digital images of breast cancer pathology and revealed that the computer algorithm achieved a predictive score strongly associated with the real-life survival rate of those studied patients (log-rank $p \le = 0.001$).

A recent study showed improvement in the mundane histopathology task of breast cancer mitotic figure counting by AI assistance [25]. Mitosis counting serves as an essential marker for breast cancer prognosis; however, it is traditionally a labor-intensive manual process. In order to discover if AI can assist in this process, a set of routinely stained slides of 320 breast ductal carcinoma cases was scanned (40 X magnification) into WSI, which was then used to train an AI algorithm to detect and count mitoses. After the computer training, 140 high-power fields of mitotic figures containing breast cancer derived from a separate dataset were used to test 24 pathologists on the task of mitosis counting with or without the assistant of AI. The results of this study illustrated that AI assistance improves both the accuracy and efficiency of mitosis counting. With AI assistance, 21 readers (87.5%) increased their identification of mitoses (true positivity), and 13 readers (54.2%) reduced their counting of falsely flagged mitoses (false positivity). Moreover, AI assistance has resulted in a 27.8% overall time saving for the readers.

Another recent study also supports DL-based AI assistance for histopathology classification of liver cancers [26].

- The researchers developed a DL-based assistant, with the aim of helping physicians in differentiating two subtypes of primary liver malignancies: hepatocellular carcinoma (HCC) and cholangiocarcinoma (CC).
- The subjects were WSI images of liver excision samples, formalin fixed, paraffin-embedded, H&E stained, scanned (at 40 X magnification), and digitalized (at 0.25 μm per pixel). Specimens

containing both HCC and CC, as well as poor quality specimens, were excluded. The dataset for training, tuning, and validation was obtained from the WSI collections (35 HCC, 35 CC) of the Cancer Genome Atlas (TCGA) data source, whereas the dataset (40 HCC, 40 CC, from 80 different patients) for independent testing was provided by the slide archives of the department of pathology at Stanford University Medical Center, and the correct diagnoses were verified by a group of histopathologists through an intradepartmental consensus review process. After randomly dividing the dataset from the TCGA and ensuring a 50:50 distribution of HCC:CC in each subset, the researchers acquired the model parameter from the training subset (20 WSI), then chose hyper-parameters with the tuning subset (24 WSI), and finally determined the generalization ability of the model with the validating subset (26 WSI).

- The model has a specific architecture of a densely connected convoluted neural network (CNN), characterized by each layer being connected to every other layer in the network, fashioning in a feed-forward manner. To accommodate the capacity of CNN, WSI was divided into patches, which contained an image size of 512 × 512 pixels and a total of 20,000 patches (1,000 patches/WSI), 2,400 patches (100 patches/WSI), and 2,600 patches (100 patches/WSI) of images were normalized (with the mean and standard deviation of pixel value in the TCGA data source) and then utilized for the training, tuning, and validating steps, respectively. At the validating step, the model achieved a diagnostic accuracy of 0.885 with a 95% confidence interval at 0.71–0.96. For the independent test, the model achieved an accuracy of 0.842 with a 95% confidence interval at 0.808–0.876.

- To assess the pathologists' accuracy with and without AI assistance, each of the 11 participants with various levels of experience in liver cancer diagnostics was assigned to read the 80 independent test WSI images twice in the same sequence. For the first reading, each read the first 40 images with AI assistance and the other 40 images without assistance; for the second reading (2 weeks or longer after the first reading), each reversed the assistance by reading the first 40 images without AI assistance and the other 40 images with assistance. The AI assistance came in a form of binary probability (HCC or CC) using a threshold of 0.5.

- This study's results revealed that the 11 pathologists as a group achieved an accuracy of 0.898 (95% confidence interval 0.875–0.916) without AI assistance and 0.914 (95% confidence interval 0.893–0.930) with AI assistance. Although for the entire group of pathologists, AI assistance improvement was not statistically significant (p = 0.184), a focused analysis did show that AI assistance provided a statistically significant improvement (p = 0.045) for a subgroup (9/11) of pathologists who had levels of well-defined pathology reading experience (three GI specialists with three or more years of diagnosis for HCC and CC, three non–GI specialists with 16 to 29 years of practice, and three trainees with HCC and CC diagnostic exposure.)

- The outcome of this model suggests that AI assistance could enhance pathologists' diagnostic accuracy, rather than replace pathologists.

Furthermore, another AI algorithm was shown to be accurate in making prostate cancer diagnosis from needle-biopsy samples in this 2020 publication [27].

- The subjects for the study were prostate tissues obtained from core needle biopsy (CNB), and the samples were placed on glass slides, stained with H & E, scanned with a Philips scanner, and digitalized.
- 549 slide samples were extracted to form 1,357,480 image patches as a training dataset, and an additional 2,501 slides were used as an internal test dataset. The subsequent validation was conducted with an external dataset of 100 consecutive clinical cases composed of 1,627 slides. Three senior pathologists (with 20 to 40 years of experience) conducted the annotations.
- The AI algorithm, developed based on multilayered CNNs, was trained on cancer detection and trained with knowledges of Gleason probability scores (high-grade 7–10, atypical small acinar proliferation grade 6), Gleason pattern 5 (for aggressive cancer), peri-neural invasion, and percent cancer present in CNB calculation.
- The researchers, upon the training, assessed the accuracy of the AI algorithm in detecting cancer.
- In the internal test, the AI algorithm achieved an area under the receiver operating characteristic curve (AUC) of 0.997 (95% confidence interval 0.995–0.998), and in the external test, the AI algorithm obtained AUC of 0.991 (95% confidence interval 0.979–1.00), indicating very high accuracy.
- The AI algorithm also achieved an AUC of 0.941 (95% confidence interval 0.905–0.977) for distinguishing high-grade prostate cancers (grade 7–10) from low-grade ones (grade 6) and an AUC of 0.971 (95% confidence interval 0.943–0.998) and an AUC of 0.957 (95% confidence interval 0.930–0.985) for detecting Gleason pattern 5 and peri-neural invasion, respectively. Moreover, the AI algorithm showed good agreement with pathologists in calculating the percent of cancer present in CNB (r = 0.882, 95% confidence interval 0.834–0.915; p < 0.0001, mean bias −4.14%).

- Importantly, the deployment of the AI algorithm as a "second-read" mechanism in real clinical practice has led to high-grade alerts on about 10% of cases diagnosed by pathologists, resulting in additional tissue sample sectioning for staining and the subsequent correct determination of one missed case of cancer initially misdiagnosed as a benign lesion by the pathologist.

UNFINISHED BUSINESS

What additional efforts do we need before AI-assisted cutaneous histopathology could become a viable clinical operation?

Major Technical Challenges and Opportunities

Recently, experts in the field of AI-assisted digital pathology have posted a list of challenges facing this area of development, as well some possible solutions for overcoming these obstacles [10]:

- *Labeled data deficiency*: An AI algorithm, if successful, needs lots of good-quality images for its training and validation processes. Not only is that large dataset needed, but these images also need to be labeled by histopathology experts. This manual labeling process, which is very labor intensive, is essential for the identification of regions of interest within the large scanned images. The obstacles include the time and financial burden for the expert physicians, suboptimal scanned image quality, constraint of network speed, and feature ambiguity. One possible solution suggested by the field experts is the utilization of unsupervised learning, which does not require labeling and would extract features without supervision.
- *Tissue variability*: The body has multiple types of tissues (neural, muscular, connective, and epithelial), and each has multiple presentation patterns, thus producing a nearly infinite number of patterns, a huge challenge from a AI computational perspective.
- *Extreme simplicity approach*: The many AI-assisted histopathology methods are simply binary in nature (e.g., yes or no, or malignant or benign). This does not take into account the conventional thought process of histopathology: clinical context understanding, perception, personal experience, and cognition. This binary decision

approach will not be applicable for difficult and rare disease cases, which are often encountered in real-life medical practice.

- *Obstacle in dimensionality*: Whole slide imaging (WSI) commonly generates a huge data dimension, like 50,000 by 50,000 pixels. Most deep ANN algorithms, on the other hand, process images with much smaller dimensions of less than 350 by 350 pixels. This poses a huge capacity challenge. One possible solution is called "patching": dividing images into many small tiles. Even with patching, down-sample (a process of pixel reduction) may be needed, and this process may result in the loss of information critical for the diagnosis.

- *Dilemma of Turing test*: Alan Turing was one of the pioneers of AI concept development. Since the principle of the Turing test states that human experts (pathologists in this case) should always be the ultimate evaluators if AI is utilized in practice (pathology in this case), full automation of AI-assisted histopathology will be either unwise or impossible. It might as well be this way. The experts in the field also support the notion that pathologists should be central not only for the development of the algorithm, but also for the execution of the algorithm.

- *Weakness of AI in uni-task approach*: The currently applied AI-assisted histopathology applications are in the category of "weak AI," meaning that they are capable of performing simple and specific tasks one at a time. The result is that major human effort is needed for the training of each and every individual task. One possible solution is "transfer learning," a process of retraining a pre-trained network for a different purpose.

- *Cost of technology*: The process of training and utilizing a DL-type AI algorithm for pixel-based data, as in histopathology, requires a high-performing graphical processing unit and highly specialized electronic circuits. In addition, the acquisition of digital histopathology needs a high capacity of computer storage. Both of these requirements pose a tremendous financial burden on a pathology department implementing AI-assisted histopathology.

- *Misleading by "adversarial attacks"*: A few publications have pointed out that "adversarial attack," a process of target manipulation of a very small number of pixels in an image, can mislead a heavy-duty deep neural network. This finding raises the possibility that the minimum noise or artifacts sometimes present in histopathology preparation, such as crushed cells, debris, contamination, or tissue folds, can be mistakenly diagnosed as cancer by AI.

- *Transparency and interpretability roadblocks*: Up to the present, we still do not understand the rationale behind the AI decision-making process, even as millions of additions and multiplications are ongoing inside a DL neural network to come up with an output (a diagnosis). Since physicians need underlying reasoning to justify a diagnostic decision, this lack of clear AI rationale becomes unacceptable for their medical practice and for approval by regulatory agencies. The experts in the field suggest the possible use of "computer vision," a conventional method that is understood and interpretable by physicians.

- *Realism for AI*: Current optimism for AI-assisted histopathology notwithstanding, realistic applications in the future depend on three key factors: 1) user friendliness (a factor of simple demands for pre-imaging effort, uncertain input, and output that is generalizable, scalable, and understandable); 2) justifiable cost effectiveness (a return of investment factor); and 3) pathologists' confidence (a physician trust factor).

Physician Perspectives

A significant survey published in 2019 illustrates concerns among physicians about the integration of AI into diagnostic pathology [14]. The subjects of this widely distributed international survey comprised 487 pathologists from 54 different countries. The participants included academic pathologists, practicing pathologists, and trainees. Although more than 70% of survey participants responded with interest in (41.2%) or excitement about (32.1%) involving AI in diagnostic pathology to improve quality assurance and workflow efficiency, a number of participants raised concerns about AI, including potential job displacement (19.7%). Overall, 51% of surveyed pathologists believed that patients would not have opinion on AI involvement in pathology diagnosis, and 29% of pathologists thought that patients would be excited about AI in the diagnostic process. Concerns about the technology barrier and AI errors were also raised by the participants; only a small percentage had no concern about AI-related error (24.8%) or believed AI errors would be lower than physicians' (10%). Most importantly, a significant number of pathologists thought that diagnostic decisions should either remain primarily a physician's responsibility (48.3%) or be an equally shared responsibility between AI and physicians (25.3%).

Trust of Cutaneous Histopathologists

A survey conducted in 2016 and responded to by 207 US dermatopathologists who perform diagnostic tasks for melanocytic lesions revealed that although most pathology participants agreed that digital WSI could be used to make correct pathology diagnosis and that WSI's benefits outweighed concerns, most participants did not have experience with WSI (59%) and did not plan to adopt it for use in the future (51%). Those who utilized it did so primarily for teaching, board exam, and continuing medical education (CME) purposes rather than for their daily practice. The majority of the respondents felt that WSI was too slow for their routine daily use. It is not known if the addition of AI to the equation would change their perception [28, 29].

The Trust of Patients

A trusting relationship between patients and their physicians is vitally important for medicine, as such a relationship will enhance treatment adherence, self-reported health improvement, and the overall patient experience [30]. If the diagnosis is determined in part by AI, would the patients trust the result? A recent survey revealed that 51% of surveyed pathologists believed that patients would not have opinion on AI involvement in histopathology diagnosis [14]. But that opinion has not been confirmed by a widely applicable study on patients' attitude toward the use of AI in medicine. Furthermore, how much of a role AI plays in histopathology diagnosis—whether it is an assistant role or a decision-making role—may determine how patients feel about AI in medicine. Some academicians argued that there are three keys for building such a trusting relationship: competency (AI's ability to enhance physicians' clinical abilities), motive (physicians' acting solely in patients' interest), and transparency (decisions based on documented evidence and expert consensus). When AI is used in medical decision making, physicians need to be informed about the source of the data and the qualification of the AI-based recommendation, and the information should be explainable. The AI knowledges will go a long way toward building a strong and trusting physician-patient relationship [30]. A critical issue involving AI is that, commonly, AI algorithms operate in a manner resembling a "black box," which provides data without detailed explanation. In addition, most physicians are not expected to be experts in AI operation. Thus, an explainable AI algorithm would be difficult to achieve [31].

Medical-Legal Consideration

If the diagnosis is aided by AI, who is responsible for the diagnostic call [32]? Does the ultimate responsibility rest on the machine or the physician who sends the patient's samples to be evaluated by the machine? Across history, physicians have utilized a variety of forms of technical assistance for diagnosis and treatment. We use radiological techniques: first simple x-rays, then later, sophisticated

CT and MRI scans. No matter how high-tech the technical assistance we have in our possession, we physicians always, with no exception, remain in the position of final decision maker. It is prudent to make sure that the physician—in this case, the pathologist—remains the final decision maker, even with the high-tech assistance of AI, as the physician will be ultimately responsible for the outcome of their patients. Some academicians argue that, in addition to demonstrating their accuracy, AI systems should also be evaluated on outcomes and on other legal criteria and undergo rigorous trials with public deliberation [33].

SUMMARY

The rapid development of AI algorithm and digital pathology over the last ten years or so has allowed the medical community to assess the viability of the AI-assisted diagnosis paradigm with digital pathology. From the analysis of recent medical publications, AI has shown its potential to help make histopathology a better diagnostic tool. Whereas some study results showed AI being superior to pathologists, others revealed that AI could improve pathologists' diagnostic accuracy and speed. While AI technology will continue to improve, more effort will be needed to address other non-technical issues such as medical-legal matters, patients' trust concern, and physicians' perspectives. Figure 3.1 illustrates a scheme for AI-assisted histopathology diagnosis for melanoma.

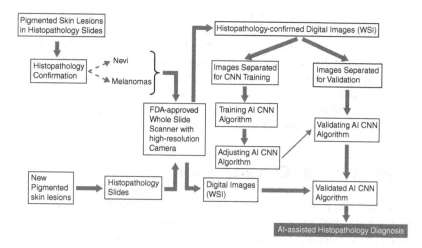

FIGURE 3.1   Schematic diagram of an AI-assisted histopathology diagnosis for pigmented skin lesions. (AI = artificial intelligence; CNN = convoluted neural network.)

REFERENCES

1. [LEXICO] Pathology. Definition of pathology in English. [www.lexico.com/en/definition/pathology] Accessed July 31,2020.
2. Riedl E, Asgari M, Alvarez D, Margaritescu I, and Gottlieb GJ. A study assessing the feasibility and diagnostic accuracy of real-time teledermatopathology. *Dermatol Pract Concept* 2012; 2(2): 0202a02. Doi: 10.5826/dpc.0202a02.
3. Parwani AV. Next generation diagnostic pathology: Use of digital pathology and artificial intelligence tools to augment a pathological diagnosis. *Diagnostic Pathol* 2019; 14: 138. https://doi.org/10.1186/s13000-019-0921-2.
4. Lever WF. *Histopathology of the Skin.* 3rd Ed. J.B. Lippincott Co., Philadelphia, 1961.
5. Lever WF. Contemporaries: Walter F. Lever, M.D. *J Am Acad Dermatol* 1984; 10(2): 321–325.
6. [ABD]. American board of dermatology. [https://abderm.org] Accessed May 20, 2020.
7. Calonje E, Brenn T, Lazar AJ, and Billings SD. *McKee's Pathology of the Skin.* 5th Ed. Elsevier, London, UK, 2019.
8. [GOOD READS]. Yann Martel, Canadian author. [goodreads.com/author/show/811.Yann_Martel] Accessed May 20, 2020.
9. Bera K, Schalper KA, Rimm DL, Velcheti V, and Madabhushi A. Artificial intelligence in digital pathology—new tools for diagnosis and precision oncology. *Nat Rev Clin Oncol* 2019; 16(11): 703–715. Doi: 10.1038/s41571-019-0252-y.
10. Tizhoosh HR and Pantanowitz L. Artificial intelligence and digital pathology: Challenges and opportunities. *J Pathol Inform* 2018; 9: 38. Doi: 10.4103/jpi.jpi_53_18.
11. Chang HY, Jung CK, Woo JI, Lee S, Cho J, Kim SW, and Kwak TY. Artificial intelligence in pathology. *J Pathol Transl Med* 2019; 53(1). Doi: 10.4132/jptm.2018.12.16.
12. Nir G, Karimi D, Goldenberg SL, Fazli L, Skinnider BF, Tavassoli P, Turbin D, et al. Comparison of artificial intelligence techniques to evaluate performance of a classifier for automatic grading of prostate cancer from digitized histopathologic images. *JAMA Netw Open* 2019; 2(3): e190442. Doi: 10.1001/jamanetworkoepn.2019.0442.
13. Rashidi HH, Tran NK, Betts EV, Howell LP, and Green R. Artificial intelligence and machine learning in pathology: The present landscape of supervised methods. *Acad Pathol* 2019; 6: 2374289519873088. Doi: 10.1177/2374289519873088.
14. Sarwar S, Dent A, Faust K, Richer M, Djuric U, Van Ommeren R, and Diamandis P. Physician perspectives on integration of artificial intelligence into diagnostic pathology. *NPJ Digit Med* 2019; 2: 28. Doi: 10.1038/s41746-019-0106-0.
15. Briganti G and Le Moine O. Artificial intelligence in medicine: Today and tomorrow. *Front Med (Lausanne)* 2020; 7: 27. Doi: 10.3389/fmed.2020.00027.
16. Cohen S. *Artificial Intelligence and Deep Learning in Pathology.* Elsevier, London, UK, 2020.
17. Jiang Y, Yang M, Wang S, Li X, and Sun Y. Emerging role of deep learning-based artificial intelligence in tumor pathology. *Cancer Commun (Lond)* 2020; 40(4): 154–166. Doi: 10.1002/cac2.12012.

18. Kalra S, Tizhoosh HR, Shah S, Choi C, Damaskinos S, Safarpoor A, Shafiei S, et al. Pan-cancer diagnostic consensus through searching archival histopathology images using artificial intelligence. *NPJ Digit Med* 2020; 3: 31. Doi: 10.1038/s41746-020-0238-2.

19. Trenholm R. Photos: The history of the digital camera. *CNET.com.* November 5, 2007. [www.cnet.com/news/photos-the-history-of-the-digital-camera/] Accessed August 5, 2020.

20. [DPA] About digital pathology. Digital Pathology Association. [www.digitalpathologyassociation.org/about-digital-pathology] Accessed July 28, 2020.

21. Evans AJ, et al. US food and drug administration approval of whole slide imaging for primary diagnosis: A key milestone is reached and new questions are raised. *Arch Pathol Lab Med* 2018; 142(11): 1381–1387.

22. Bauer TW, et al. Validation of whole slide imaging for primary diagnosis in surgical pathology. *Arch Pathol Lab Med* 2013; 137(4): 518–524.

23. Amin S, Mori T, and Itoh T. A validation study of whole slide imaging for primary diagnosis of lymphoma. *Pathol Int* 2019; 69(6): 341–349.

24. Beck AH, et al. Systematic analysis of breast cancer morphology uncovers stromal eastures associated with survival. *Sci Transl Med* 2011; 3(108): 108ra113.

25. Pantanowitz L, Hartman D, Qi Y, et al. Accuracy and efficiency of an artificial intelligence tool when counting breast mitoses. *Diagnostic Pathol* 2020; 15: 80. https://doi.org/10.1186/s13000-020-00995-z.

26. Kiani A, Uyumazturk B, Rajpurkar P, et al. Impact of a deep learning assistant on the histopathologic classification of liver cancer. *NPJ Digital Med* 2020; 3: 23. https://doi.org.10.1038/s41746-020-0232-8.

27. Pantanowitz L, Quiroga-Garza GM, Bien L, et al. An artificial intelligence algorithm for prostate cancer diagnosis in whole slide images of core needle biopsies: A blinded clinical validation and deployment study. *Lancet Digital Health* 2020; 2: e407–e416.

28. Onega T, Reisch LM, Frederick PD, et al. Use of digital whoe slide imaging in dermatopathology. *J Digit Imaging* 2016; 29: 243–253. Doi 10.1007/s10278-015-9836-y.

29. Asan O, Bayrak AE, and Choudhury A. Artificial intelligence and human trust in healthcare: Focus on clinicians. *J Med Internet Res* 2020; 22(6): e15154. Doi: 10.2196/15154.

30. Nundy S, Montgomery T, and Wachter RM. Promoting trust between patients and physicians in the era of artificial intelligence. *JAMA* 2019; 322(6): 497–498. Doi: 10.1001/jama.2018.20563.

31. Triberti S, Durosini I, Gurigliano G, et al. Is explanation a marketing problem? The quest for trust in artificial intelligence and two conflicting solutions. *Public Health Genomics* 2020; 23: 2–5. Doi: 10.1159/000506014.

32. Gerke S, Minssen T, and Cohen G. Ethical and legal challenges of artificial intelligence-driven healthcare. *Artificial Intelligence in Healthcare* 2020: 295–336. Doi: 10.1016/B978-0-12-818438-7.00012-5.

33. Carter SM, Rogers W, Win KT, et al. The ethical, legal and social implications of using artificial intelligence system in breast cancer care. *The Breast* 2020; 49: 25–32. https://doi.10.1016/j.breast.2019.10.001.

Optical Coherence Tomography for Melanoma Detection

Kamran Avanaki and Peter E. Andersen

Contents

INTRODUCTION

Melanoma is the deadliest form of skin cancer. The incidence of melanoma has been rising faster than that of any other cancer, mainly due to changes in sun exposure behavior as well as climate change [1, 2]. The American Cancer Society's estimates for melanoma in the United States for 2017 are 87,110 new melanomas diagnosed; 9,730 people are expected to die of melanoma [3]. The survival rate for melanoma patients depends on the stage of the disease when

DOI: 10.1201/9781003121275-5

diagnosed; if melanoma is detected in stage I, the survival rate is more than 90%, while if detected in stage III, it drops to less than 40%.

Traditionally, in general medical care, diagnosis of melanoma starts with visual inspection of skin lesions. Visual evaluation criteria for suspected melanomas include the ABCDE criteria (asymmetry, border irregularity, color variation, diameter >6 mm, evolving) [4, 5]. Skin lesions that fulfill the ABCDE criteria are then biopsied for histopathologic analysis [6, 7]. The specificity and sensitivity (~50% to 81% [8]) of visual inspection criteria, ABCDE, vary when used singly or in combination. This wide variability is due to subjective interpretation by physicians. This results in unnecessary biopsy of many benign lesions, ranging from 15 to 30 benign lesions biopsied to diagnose one melanoma [9]. Performing biopsies can result in pain, anxiety, scarring, and disfigurement for patients. In addition, finding a malignant lesion to biopsy among many pigmented spots (e.g., freckles or benign nevi) is difficult with visual inspection. Sampling of biopsied tissue in the histology lab is limited to 2% to 5% of the sample, and there is a 30% discordance rate among histologists in challenging cases.

Several non-invasive imaging techniques have been developed to identify melanoma. Dermoscopy depends on the appearance of classic dermoscopic features [10] and therefore has limited utility in the diagnosis of very early and mainly featureless melanomas [11]. Multispectral imaging captures image data within specific wavelength ranges across the electromagnetic spectrum; this data, however, is projected on the same plane, obscuring depth information [12]. Reflectance confocal microscopy provides cellular information on melanocytic lesions; however, its penetration depth is too limited to detect invasive melanoma [13]. High-frequency ultrasound has a satisfactory penetration depth, but the low specificity precludes diagnosis of the actual type of malignancy [14]. Recently, raster scanning photoacoustic (PA) microscopy and cross-sectional PA tomography have been explored for diagnosis and staging of melanoma [15, 16], in which melanin serves as an endogenous contrast agent. However, melanin is not a tumor specific biomarker of melanoma as it is present in benign nevi and may actually be absent in amelanotic melanoma [17]. There have been several melanoma detection devices marketed such as MelaFind [18], MoleMate SIAscope [19], Verisante Aura [20], and Nevisence [20]. These devices were developed to assist clinicians with any level of experience in the detection of melanoma and subsequently rely on histopathological assessment. However, these devices suffer various drawbacks that result in limited specificity (68% [12], 77% [21], 68% [22], and 34% [23], respectively), and/or sensitivity (93% [12], 81% [21], 90% [22], and 94% [23], respectively) and are therefore of limited benefit to the clinician. More importantly, they do not provide any information other than a score or probability that determines whether to biopsy the lesion or not. In addition, none of these devices has depth discrimination capability or provides detailed subsurface structural information.

ANALYSIS OF THE NEED

Optical coherence tomography (OCT), with a high spatial resolution (<10 microns), intermediate penetration depth (~1.5 to 2 mm), and volumetric structural and vascular imaging capability has become a popular diagnostic-assistant modality in dermatology, especially for the detection and diagnosis of non-melanoma skin tumors: e.g., basal cell carcinoma (BCC) and squamous cell carcinoma (SCC) [24–30]. Moreover, OCT is an easy-to-use device that does not require extensive training (as opposed to more sophisticated methods such as confocal, two-photon, and photoacoustic imaging) and can image vasculature. Therefore, OCT images by providing morphology of the skin and angiography of the vessels, along with soma image processing and machine-learning methods can highlight the relevant diagnostic information, yielding unprecedented sensitivity/specificity.

Tissue contrast in OCT images is generated by the intrinsic characteristics that are proportional to the density, size, and shape of tissue microstructures. Extraction of tissue optical properties from OCT images is therefore a generic method for obtaining quantitative information about tissue microstructure [31]. Because malignant cells have different characteristics than benign nevi in terms of size, order, and density, according to light-tissue interaction theories, OCT images are expected to discriminate malignant tissues from healthy tissues and benign neoplasms. However, the sensitivity and specificity of OCT for melanoma detection are lower than anticipated because the radiomic features of malignant tissues versus benign nevi in OCT images are not sufficiently specific [27, 32–36]. Several groups, including ours [37], have attempted to increase specificity by image enhancement [38], texture analysis [39–44], and even implementing sophisticated configurations of OCT, including polarization-sensitive, phase-sensitive, and dynamic OCT; these have also failed to adequately discriminate between melanoma and benign lesions.

We seek to minimize these potential errors by creating a unified objective evaluation platform in which OCT will be employed along with optical radiomic melanoma detection (ORMD) protocol [45]. The ORMD protocol is applied to OCT images of the suspect lesion and will provide the clinician with clear information on the tissue status (e.g., "Tissue sample is consistent with healthy tissue"; "Tissue sample exhibits characteristics consistent with melanoma"). This algorithm will 1) reduce the number of unnecessary biopsies by helping identify the most probable malignant lesion in a person with multiple pigmented spots, which will result in fewer biopsies and less pain, anxiety, and scarring for patients; 2) considerably reduce cost to the healthcare system; and 3) detect melanoma in its early stage, when prognosis is optimal. Importantly, the optical properties come at no additional cost as they are embedded in the image data and can readily be extracted via post-processing applicable to virtually all OCT systems.

As with any technology, the clinician is the final arbiter as to the health status of the patient. Our goal is to support the clinician in making the best possible decision. The ORMD system will provide a variety of information: 1) OCT 2D and 3-D images of the tissue under investigation with comparative side-by-side of the patient's healthy tissue; 2) vascular information of the tissue region: i.e., increased blood supply is a hallmark of cancerous lesions; and 3) OCT absorption image and scattering image maps of an individual patient's healthy tissue and the suspect lesion(s). Based on the individual optical attributes disaggregated from the OCT image, the clinician will be able to visually compare morphological differences.

Optical property differences between healthy, benign nevi and melanoma tissues that translate into OCT radiomic features are 1) scattering and absorption coefficients increase with the concentration of melanocytes (healthy: 14 ± 3 %, benign nevi: $18 \pm 3\%$, melanoma: $71 \pm 11\%$); 2) anisotropy factor increases with cell size (healthy: 6 ± 0.4 μm, benign nevi: 7 ± 0.4 μm, melanoma: 16 ± 3 μm); and 3) tissue disorder increases from healthy to melanoma, due to cellular displacement [46]. Ostensibly, the aggregation of the predominant optical properties that contribute to OCT image formation diminishes the specificity of melanoma detection due to interrelationships of these properties.

Apart from the need to improve the specificity and sensitivity of OCT for early-stage melanoma detection, there is urgency to develop this methodology due to high healthcare costs. Each year in the US, approximately $1.2 billion in healthcare spending is attributed to melanoma detection and diagnosis. A recent article by Coldiron and Ratnarathorn [47] documents that, in 2012, mid-level healthcare professionals independently billed approximately 2.6 million biopsies, which required clinical distinction between benign and malignant lesions. This number is growing approximately 6% annually. Each biopsy costs a lot, inclusive of all costs, making this a large expense to healthcare and providing a large potential market for a robust system to accurately detect melanoma.

THE TECHNOLOGY: OCT FOR MELANOMA DETECTION

The light-tissue interaction specific to OCT imaging (i.e., OCT modeling) was initiated by Schmitt, who considered only scattering coefficient for modeling using the single-scattering theory (i.e., the ballistic component only) [48]. Studies have shown that the primary effect of multiple scattering is a less steep slope of signal decay with depth than predicted by the so-called single-scattering model. Since then, several other groups have considered quantitative analysis of OCT images to improve diagnosis [49–52]. The first model that adequately includes the ballistic light component and multiple scattered light is an analytical solution to the scalar wave equation based on mutual coherence functions known as the extended Huygens-Fresnel (EHF) principle. It includes diffraction effects, and it allows Gaussian beam under any focusing condition [53, 54]. We have integrated the lateral coherence length variation with depth into previous models by considering the so-called "shower curtain effect." The model describes the heterodyne OCT signal as a function of depth. This model incorporates both multiple scattering and single scattering effects. Later, we employed the EHF principle and proposed an OCT model in a multilayer-scattering geometry [44, 53]. Here, we apply a further extension to our previous model with the addition of a third parameter, absorption coefficient, to scattering coefficient and anisotropy factor [45]. The mean squared of the OCT heterodyne signal current at the probing depth z is described as: $i^2(z) = i^2{}_0 \psi_{SA}(z)$, where $i^2{}_0 = a / w_H^2$ is the mean squared heterodyne signal current in the absence of scattering and absorption, a is a constant characterized by the OCT system setup, and w_H^2 is 1/e irradiance radius at the probing depth in the absence of scattering: $w_H^2 = w_0^2(A - B/f)^2 + (B/kw_0)^2$, where A and B are the elements of ABCD matrix for light propagation from the lens plane to the probing depth in the sample. If the focal plane of the beam is fixed on the surface of the sample, then $A = 1$ and $B = f + z/n$, where n is the refractive index, and f is the focal length of the lens, w_0 represents the 1/e irradiance radius of the input sample beam at the lens plane. $k = 2\pi / \lambda$, and λ is the wavelength of light source. $\psi_{SA}(z)$ is the heterodyne efficiency factor describing signal degradation due to scattering and absorption, $\psi_{SA}(z) = e^{-2\mu_a z}[e^{-2\mu_s z}(4e^{-\mu_s z}[1 - e^{-\mu_s z}]/ (1 + \mu_a \Delta z_D)(1 + (w_{SA}^2 / w_H^2)) + (1 - e^{-\mu_s z})^2 w_H^2 / (1 - e^{-\mu_s z})^2 w_H^2 (1 + \mu_a \Delta z_D)^2 w_{SA}^2]$. The first term in the brackets represents the single scattering effect; the third term is the multiple-scattering term; and the second term is the cross term including both single and multiple scattering. $w_{SA}^2 = (1 + \mu_a \Delta z_D)^{-1}[w_0^2(A - B/f)^2 + (B/kw_0)^2 + (2B/k\rho_0)^2(1 + \mu_a \Delta z_N)]$, is the 1/e irradiance radius at the probing depth in the presence of scattering and absorption, $\rho_0 = \sqrt{(3/\mu_s z)} \, \lambda \pi \theta_{rms} \, \lambda \pi \theta_{rms}(1 + n_R d(z)/z)$. where ρ_0 is the lateral coherence length given by θ_{rms} is the root mean squared scattering angle, defined as half-width at 1/e maximum of a Gaussian curve fitted to the main frontal lobe of the scattering phase function, and n_R is the real part of refractive index. Also, Δz_N, and Δz_D are presented by

$$\Delta z_N = z(w_0^2 + \rho_0^2 / 2) / 4n_R^2 B^2 \text{ and } \Delta z_D = \frac{z}{2n_R^2}[(w_0 / f)^2 + (1/kw_0)^2 + (2/k\rho_0)^2].$$

The ORMD protocol is implemented in MATLAB2015a. The OCT images from suspect lesion and nearby healthy skin are the inputs to the OPE algorithm, which is the core of the ORMD protocol. A precise physical OCT model is used in the OPE algorithm to extract the optical properties of a tissue from a specific region of interest. The workflow of the OPE algorithm is as follows (see Figure 4.1): a region of interest is specified in an OCT B-scan image. The pixel intensities along the x-axis in each ROI are averaged to obtain an averaged A-line. Using a fitting algorithm, the scattering and absorption coefficients as well as the anisotropy factor in the modeled OCT signal are adjusted, in order to obtain a curve that best fits the averaged A-line. By repetition for several regions of interest (ROIs), which are averaged, and standard deviations calculated, we derive optical radiomic features for that tissue: mean and standard deviation of scattering and absorption coefficients and anisotropy factor. These radiomic features obtained from the suspect lesion and its nearby healthy skin are used to create a set of normalized optical radiomic features that accounts for gender, age, and skin color. For classification, we used machine-learning algorithms. Machine learning is employed as an essential part of the supervised classification between optical radiomic features of melanoma and non-melanoma. The reason we use machine learning instead of a classical statistical classifier is as follows: while we recognize that there are other valid classification methods, such as classical statistical ones, a machine-learning approach will provide the best long-term results for the widest variation of melanoma types and stages. Since the system results will be validated histologically, the system can be taught the most nuanced variations in cytology to identify melanoma from its earliest beginnings. Additionally, the a priori knowledge we have of OCT images and healthy and melanoma tissue histology allows the training of a machine-learning kernel with greater decision-making power than a comparable system using statistical classifiers. The machine learning algorithm includes two phases: 1) training phase and 2) test phase. In the training phase, the optical radiomic features and their labels (histology results) are input to a machine-learning algorithm. In the test phase, OCT images of a suspect skin area will be analyzed by the trained machine-learning kernel with the selected optical radiomic features (i.e., optical radiomic signatures) and then suggest the status of the tissue: "Tissue sample is consistent with healthy tissue," or "Tissue sample exhibits characteristics consistent with melanoma."

UNFINISHED BUSINESS

There are many parameters in different stages of ORMD protocol. To ensure the algorithm is working at its highest possible efficiency, all combinations of

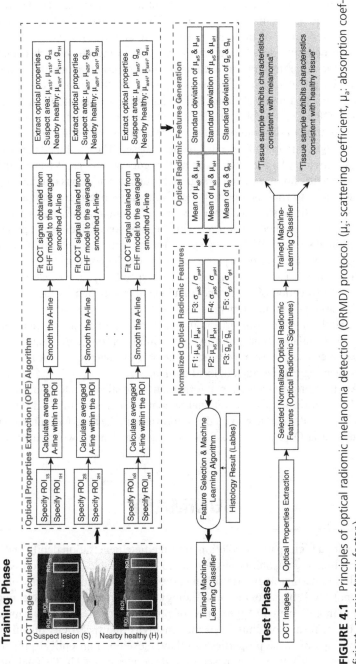

FIGURE 4.1 Principles of optical radiomic melanoma detection (ORMD) protocol. (μ_s: scattering coefficient, μ_a: absorption coefficient, g: anisotropy factor.)

parameters need to be assessed: this is the optimization process. In our preliminary work [45], parameters were selected based on individual performance; we optimized some of these parameters individually. However, in order to reach the optimum set of parameters, we plan to search through combinations of these parameters and eventually find the combination that achieves the highest possible specificity and sensitivity for the correct identification of melanoma and non-melanoma. These parameters originate from different stages of ORMD protocol, including OCT image acquisition, pre-processing, OPE algorithm, optical radiomic feature generation procedure, and machine-learning algorithm in both training and test phases. The combined parameters form an extremely large search space on the order of billions. When a problem gets sufficiently large, we need to search through an enormous number of possible solutions to find the optimal one. Even with modern computing power, finding the optimal solution is not possible on a human timescale. Therefore, an optimization method is required, with the intention of finding an optimal or near-optimal solution. We have two goals for this optimization task: 1) achieve the highest possible sensitivity (true positive) for the correct identification of melanoma and 2) achieve the highest possible specificity (true negative) for the correct identification of benign nevi and healthy. This makes the problem a two-dimensional optimization process. Due to the very large size of the search space and the non-linear nature of our optimization problem, we are planning to use the simulated annealing (SA) algorithm to optimize the search for the best parameter set. The main characteristic of SA is that the algorithm is excellent at avoiding getting stuck in local optima.

Angiography is more free information concealed in OCT images. We intend to investigate this as additional radiomic features for the ORMD protocol to improve its accuracy. With this improvement, the need for multimodality devices such as OCT/photoacoustic to investigate melanoma will be eliminated.

SUMMARY

OCT, with a high spatial resolution, intermediate penetration depth, and volumetric imaging capability has proven to be a valuable diagnostic-assistant modality in dermatology. At this time, the sensitivity and specificity of conventional OCT by assessing morphology only for melanoma detection is lower than anticipated. Aggregation of optical properties that contribute to OCT image formation diminishes the sensitivity and specificity due to interrelationships of these properties. We have developed an optical properties extraction (OPE) algorithm, based on a three-parameter OCT signal model (patent pending), to disaggregate the OCT image into its individual optical attributes (i.e., scattering and absorption coefficients and anisotropy factor), which correlate to tissue architecture (i.e., cell number, size, shape, and disorder). Optical radiomic features are calculated from the optical properties and input to a supervised machine-learning algorithm; the trained kernel then will be used for differentiation of melanoma from non-melanoma. This is the basis of our optical radiomic melanoma detection (ORMD) protocol. The protocol has been tested on OCT images of more than 100 human subjects and differentiated melanoma from benign nevi with 96% sensitivity and 95% specificity.

REFERENCES

1. Linos E, et al. Increasing burden of melanoma in the United States. *Journal of Investigative Dermatology* 2009; 129(7): 1666–1674.
2. Bharath A and Turner R. Impact of climate change on skin cancer. *Journal of the Royal Society of Medicine* 2009; 102(6): 215–218.
3. Key Statistics for Melanoma Skin Cancer. 2017. [www.cancer.org/cancer/melanoma-skin-cancer/about/key-statistics.html].
4. Friedman RJ, Rigel DS, and Kopf AW. Early detection of malignant melanoma: The role of physician examination and self-examination of the skin. *CA: A Cancer Journal for Clinicians* 1985; 35(3): 130–151.
5. MacKie RM. Clinical recognition of early invasive malignant melanoma. *BMJ: British Medical Journal* 1990; 301(6759): 1005.
6. Orchard G. Comparison of immunohistochemical labelling of melanocyte differentiation antibodies melan-A, tyrosinase and HMB 45 with NKIC3 and S100 protein in the evaluation of benign naevi and malignant melanoma. *The Histochemical Journal* 2000; 32(8): 475–481.
7. Snyder ML and Paulino AF. Melan-A as a useful diagnostic immunohistochemical stain for the diagnosis of primary sinonasal melanomas. *Head & Neck* 2002; 24(1): 52–55.
8. Thomas L, et al. Semiological value of ABCDE criteria in the diagnosis of cutaneous pigmented tumors. *Dermatology* 1998; 197(1): 11–17.
9. Wilson RL, et al. How good are US dermatologists at discriminating skin cancers? A number-needed-to-treat analysis. *Journal of Dermatological Treatment* 2012; 23(1): 65–69.
10. Arpaia N, Cassano N, and Vena GA. Dermoscopic patterns of dermatofibroma. *Dermatologic Surgery* 2005; 31(10): 1336–1339.
11. Skvara H, et al. Limitations of dermoscopy in the recognition of melanoma. *Archives of Dermatology* 2005; 141(2): 155–160.
12. Elbaum M, et al. Automatic differentiation of melanoma from melanocytic nevi with multispectral digital dermoscopy: A feasibility study. *Journal of the American Academy of Dermatology* 2001; 44(2): 207–218.

13. Pellacani G, et al. The impact of in vivo reflectance confocal microscopy for the diagnostic accuracy of melanoma and equivocal melanocytic lesions. *Journal of Investigative Dermatology* 2007; 127(12): 2759–2765.
14. Frinking PJ, et al. Ultrasound contrast imaging: Current and new potential methods. *Ultrasound in Medicine & Biology* 2000; 26(6): 965–975.
15. Oh JT, et al. Three-dimensional imaging of skin melanoma in vivo by dual-wavelength photoacoustic microscopy. *Journal of Biomedical Optics* 2006; 11(3): 034032.
16. Zhou Y, et al. Noninvasive determination of melanoma depth using a handheld photoacoustic probe. *The Journal of Investigative Dermatology* 2017; 137(6): 1370.
17. Zelickson AS. The fine structure of the human melanotic and amelanotic malignant melanoma. *Journal of Investigative Dermatology* 1962; 39(6): 605–613.
18. Monheit G, et al. The performance of MelaFind: A prospective multicenter study. *Archives of Dermatology* 2011; 147(2): 188–194.
19. Michalska M, Chodorowska G, and Krasowska D. SIAscopy—a new non-invasive technique of melanoma diagnosis. *Annales Universitatis Mariae Curie-Sklodowska. Sectio D: Medicina* 2004; 59(2): 421–431.
20. Fink C and Haenssle H. Non-invasive tools for the diagnosis of cutaneous melanoma. *Skin Research and Technology* 2017; 23(3): 261–271.
21. Tomatis S, et al. Automated melanoma detection with a novel multispectral imaging system: Results of a prospective study. *Physics in Medicine & Biology* 2005; 50(8): 1675.
22. Lui H, et al. Real-time Raman spectroscopy for in vivo skin cancer diagnosis. *Cancer Research* 2012: p. canres. 4061.2011.
23. Malvehy J, et al. Clinical performance of the nevisense system in cutaneous melanoma detection: An international, multicentre, prospective and blinded clinical trial on efficacy and safety. *British Journal of Dermatology* 2014; 171(5): 1099–1107.
24. Coleman AJ, et al. Histological correlates of optical coherence tomography in non-melanoma skin cancer. *Skin Research and Technology* 2013; 19(1): e10–e19.
25. Alawi SA, et al. Optical coherence tomography for presurgical margin assessment of non-melanoma skin cancer—a practical approach. *Exp Dermatol* 2013; 22(8): 547–551.
26. Mogensen M, et al. Assessment of optical coherence tomography imaging in the diagnosis of non-melanoma skin cancer and benign lesions versus normal skin: Observer-blinded evaluation by dermatologists and pathologists. *Dermatologic Surgery* 2009; 35(6): 965–972.
27. Fercher AF. Optical coherence tomography—development, principles, applications. *Z Med Phys* 2010; 20(4): 251–276.
28. Welzel J, et al. Optical coherence tomography of the human skin. *J Am Acad Dermatol* 1997; 37(6): 958–963.
29. Steiner R, Kunzi-Rapp K, and Scharffetter-Kochanek K. Optical coherence tomography: Clinical applications in dermatology. *Medical Laser Application* 2003; 18(3): 249–259.
30. Pierce MC, et al. Advances in optical coherence tomography imaging for dermatology. *J Invest Dermatol* 2004; 123(3): 458–463.
31. Chang S and Bowden AK. Review of methods and applications of attenuation coefficient measurements with optical coherence tomography. *Journal of Biomedical Optics* 2019; 24(9): 090901.

32. Gambichler T, et al. Applications of optical coherence tomography in dermatology. *J Dermatol Sci* 2005; 40(2): 85–94.
33. Holmes J and Welzel J. OCT in dermatology. *Optical Coherence Tomography: Technology and Applications* 2015: 2189–2207.
34. Sattler E, Kästle R, and Welzel J. Optical coherence tomography in dermatology. *Journal of Biomedical Optics* 2013; 18(6): 061224.
35. Welzel J. Optical coherence tomography in dermatology: A review. *Skin Research and Technology* 2001; 7(1): 1–9.
36. Zysk AM, et al. Optical coherence tomography: A review of clinical development from bench to bedside. *Journal of Biomedical Optics* 2007; 12(5): 051403–051421.
37. Adabi S, et al. Universal in vivo textural model for human skin based on optical coherence tomograms. *Scientific Reports* 2017; 7(1): 17912.
38. Adabi S, et al. An overview of methods to mitigate artifacts in optical coherence tomography imaging of the skin. *Skin Research and Technology* 2018; 24(2): 265–273.
39. Pentland AP. Fractal-based description of natural scenes. *IEEE Transactions on Pattern Analysis and Machine Intelligence* 1984(6): 661–674.
40. Amadasun M and King R. Textural features corresponding to textural properties. *IEEE Transactions on Systems, Man, and Cybernetics* 1989; 19(5): 1264–1274.
41. Thibault G, Angulo J, and Meyer F. Advanced statistical matrices for texture characterization: Application to cell classification. *IEEE Transactions on Biomedical Engineering* 2014; 61(3): 630–637.
42. Galloway MM. Texture analysis using gray level run lengths. *Computer Graphics and Image Processing* 1975; 4(2): 172–179.
43. Adabi S, et al. Textural analysis of optical coherence tomography skin images: Quantitative differentiation between healthy and cancerous tissues. *Progress in Biomedical Optics and Imaging* 2017; 10053: 100533F.
44. Levitz D, et al. Determination of optical scattering properties of highly-scattering media in optical coherence tomography images. *Optics Express* 2004; 12(2): 249–259.
45. Turani Z, et al. Optical radiomic signatures derived from optical coherence tomography images improve identification of melanoma. *Cancer Research* 2019; 79(8): 2021–2030.
46. Available from: http://omlc.org/calc/mie_calc.html.
47. Coldiron B and Ratnarathorn M. Scope of physician procedures independently billed by mid-level providers in the office setting. *JAMA Dermatology* 2014; 150(11): 1153–1159.
48. Schmitt JM, et al. Optical-coherence tomography of a dense tissue: Statistics of attenuation and backscattering. *Physics in Medicine and Biology* 1994; 39(10): 1705.
49. Adegun OK, et al. Quantitative analysis of optical coherence tomography and histopathology images of normal and dysplastic oral mucosal tissues. *Lasers in Medical Science* 2012; 27(4): 795–804.
50. Kubo T, et al. Plaque and thrombus evaluation by optical coherence tomography. *The International Journal of Cardiovascular Imaging* 2011; 27(2): 289–298.
51. Zhang Q, et al. Quantitative analysis of rectal cancer by spectral domain optical coherence tomography. *Physics in Medicine & Biology* 2012; 57(16): 5235.

52. Avanaki MR, et al. Quantitative evaluation of scattering in optical coherence tomography skin images using the extended huygens-fresnel theorem. *Applied Optics* 2013; 52(8): 1574–1580.
53. Thrane L, Yura HT, and Andersen PE. Analysis of optical coherence tomography systems based on the extended huygens-fresnel principle. *JOSA A* 2000; 17(3): 484–490.
54. Yura HT, Thrane L, and Andersen PE. Closed-form solution for the Wigner phase-space distribution function for diffuse reflection and small-angle scattering in a random medium. *JOSA A* 2000; 17(12): 2464–2474.

PART II

Regenerative Cutaneous Medicine

Regeneration of Human Hair Follicles by 3-D Bioprinting

5

Lawrence S. Chan

Contents

DOI: 10.1201/9781003121275-7

INTRODUCTION

Bioprinting Defined

Before we go into the detailed discussion of 3-D bioprinting as a regenerative medical methodology, a clear definition of 3-D bioprinting is in order. But even before that, we should first clarify what 3-D printing is. *Merriam-Webster's Dictionary* defines 3-D printing as "the manufacturing of solid objects by the deposition of layers of material (such as plastic) in accordance with specifications that are stored and displayed in electronic form as a digital model" [1]. In industrial terms, it is also referred as "additive manufacturing." While 3-D printing has been in industrial use for some time, 3-D bioprinting is a relatively new undertaking, and this term cannot be found in *Merriam-Webster's Dictionary* as of April 2020 [1]. A biomedical publication in 2018 stated it this way:

> Bioprinting is an emerging field in regenerative medicine. Producing cell-laden, three-dimensional structures to mimic bodily tissues has an important role not only in tissue engineering, but also in drug delivery and cancer studies. Bioprinting can provide patient-specific spatial geometry, controlled microstructures and the positioning of different cell types for the fabrication of tissue engineering scaffolds [2].

In other words, 3-D bioprinting is the biological counterpart of industrial 3-D printing, fabricating biologically compatible solid tissues that mimic the functions of natural biological tissues. Although on the surface there seems to be a small difference between 3-D printing and 3-D bioprinting, the jump is actually very substantial, as one is a non-viable product, and the other is a living tissue. Thus, one of the biggest challenges for the bioprinting process is how to keep the cells viable during the "printing" process and how to layer the live cells along with other essential biological components in a nature-mimicking way so that the finished product will actually provide a living environment and biologically compatible functions. Without a viable functionality, the bioengineered tissue simply cannot restore the biological functions we seek. In this chapter, the bioengineered human hair follicle will be discussed. First, some technical details and the advantages and disadvantages of bioprinting methods will be described, as there are three types of bioprinting fabrication methods: laser based, extrusion based, and inkjet based. Then, the need for bioengineering hair is discussed, followed by step-by-step detailing of a successful prototype of a human hair follicle. Finally, the additional work needed to make this type of hair follicle a successful commercial product will be delineated.

Inkjet-Based Method

The first method developed for bioprinting, the inkjet-based technique utilizes a commercially available inkjet printer specially adapted to print the biological materials (bioink). The initial problem of sample drying was later corrected by developing the cell-loaded hydrogel to encapsulate the bioink from drying. In a nutshell, inkjet bioprinting forms the intended cells and biomaterials into a desirable pattern in droplets and then ejects these fluid mixtures through a micro-nozzle onto scaffold platforms by one of two processes: the thermal process or the piezoelectric process. The first process relies on heat-induced bubble nucleation to propel bioink through the micro-nozzle; the second process utilizes an actuator that produces an acoustic wave to propel the bioink through the micro-nozzle. Although the temperature of the heating element in the thermal process can reach as high as 300^{0}C, the localized effect of short heat duration does not result in significant cellular damages. Inkjet bioprinters have the advantages of excellent resolution (up to 50 µm), high speed, low cost, excellent cell viability, and wide availability but have the disadvantage of low droplet directionality and unreliable cell encapsulation. One of the shortcomings of piezoelectric process, on the other hand, is its operational limitation on high-concentration or high-viscosity bioink [2].

Extrusion-Based Method

A similar method that also utilizes a micro-nozzle to lay bioink on scaffold platforms is extrusion-based bioprinting. The extrusion of bioink is a pressure-driven process utilizing either air (pneumatic) or mechanical (piston) pressure. The superior aspect of this method is the ability to print materials with high cellular density. The limitation of this method is a relatively low resolution of around 100 µm, which is not suitable for applications requiring small pore sizes (<10 mm), lacking the ability for cell positioning, potential alteration of cell morphology and function by extrusion pressure, and the potential of induced cell apoptosis in highly viscous hydrogel. The latter limitation is due to the fact that the higher viscosity induces a greater shear stress, which is directly linked to cell apoptotic activity [2].

Laser-Based Method

This third method of bioprinting, also termed stereolithography, is based on the principle of polymerization by light energy, commonly derived from UV light or visible light and offers a resolution ranging from 5 to 300 μm. Unlike the two previously discussed methods, this method is a nozzle-free technique. After a layer of fluid monomeric bioink is loaded onto a scaffold platform, light energy is applied to induce the polymerization of the platform-loaded bioink, and then the platform is lowered to accept the next layer of bioink. The process continues until all layers of bioink are loaded and polymerized. Since this is a photopolymerization process, it requires a photosensitizing chemical (photo-initiator) to induce the polymerization: that is, to make the polymer photosensitive in response to light. Two commonly used and least toxic photo-initiators are "eosin Y" (crosslinking monomers to form polymers at visible light wave length 400–700 nm) and "Irgacure 2959" (crosslinking monomers at UV wave length). The major advantage of this laser-based method is the total elimination of the negative effects of pressure and shear stress induced by nozzle-based techniques, good resolution, unlimited bioink viscosity, speed, and accuracy. The less-than-desirable aspects of this method are the potential toxicity of the photosensitizer and the potential mutational effect of UV light if it is the chosen light source. As eosin Y has been shown to be less toxic and visible light is less likely to induce cellular mutation, the current trend in the laser-based method is toward eosin Y and other visible light photo-initiators, and research is ongoing to hunt for a method that eliminates photo-initiators altogether. The laser-assisted method will be discussed in greater details elsewhere [2].

ANALYSIS Of THE NEED

Any entrepreneur who wants to start a new line of products must do an analysis to determine how viable the new product will be. One of the commonly used methodologies for pre-marketing study is called the SWOT (strength, weakness, opportunities, and threats) analysis [3, 4]. For obvious reasons, a product that has the potential to fill an unmet need will have a greater chance of success than one with which the market is already saturated. Therefore, the need for manufacturing human hair follicles will now be examined.

Alopecia (hair loss) is a cutaneous problem that affects many patients. Although it is not a life-threatening condition, it affects patients' social function and mental health significantly. Alopecia has many types. Some are genetically programmed; others are immune mediated, inflammatory, or autoimmune in nature [5]. The genetically programmed hair thinning, usually referred as male- or female-pattern (androgenetic) alopecia, is one of the most common chronic problems encountered by dermatologists [6, 7]. The major autoimmune-mediated alopecia forms include alopecia areata (a patchy form of hair loss) and the more extensive forms of alopecia totalis and alopecia universalis. A loss of hair follicle "immune privilege" is thought to be the trigger for the development of the alopecia areata group of diseases [8]. Androgenetic alopecia and alopecia areata groups, the most prevalent non-scarring forms of hair loss disorders with their follicles intact, are characterized by rapidly cycling miniaturizing hair follicles that fail to form quality terminal hairs. Other forms of inflammatory alopecia that tends to result in scarring include lichen planopilaris, frontal fibrosing alopecia, lupus-related alopecia, acne keloidalis nuchae, central centrifugal cicatricial alopecia, Brocq pseudopelade, folliculitis decalvans, dissecting folliculitis, and Brunsting-Perry cicatricial pemphigoid of the scalp [9, 10]. Medical treatments can help restore the lost hair in certain types of the alopecia with varying degrees of success but cannot help patients who develop scarring forms of alopecia restore lost hair.

Since some forms of alopecia tend to affect young people during an important time of their lives for courtship, the negative psychological impact on the patients can be very profound. Just for alopecia areata alone, the global DALYs (disability-adjusted life years), a term measuring disease burden, were calculated to be 1,332,800 in 2010, with patients at risk for co-morbidities of depression, anxiety, and other psychological conditions [11]. Alopecia areata has an estimated incidence of 20 per 100,000 person-years with a lifetime incidence of 2%, and it accounts for 25% of all types of alopecia [12–14]. A quality-of-life study of 200 patients with androgenetic alopecia revealed that these patients have a DLQI (dermatology life quality index) mean score of 13.52 (out of maximum best score of 30), pointing to an important quality of life issue [7]. For obvious reasons, alopecia has greater negative impact on female patients than on their male counterparts [15]. This importance of hair to quality of life was vividly stated by a famous American actress, Joan Crawford: "I think that the most important thing a woman can have—next to talent, of course—is her hairdresser" [16]. Arguably, from the perspective of its highly negative impact on patients' mental health, alopecia should be treated as a medical condition rather than a cosmetic concern [8].

For androgenetic alopecia, which affects more than 50% of men over the age of 50 and 13% of premenopausal women, the available treatments include medical and surgical types [10, 17]. The medical treatments include topical minoxidil solution, which does provide some success, but continuous life-long treatment is required to maintain the success [17]. In fact, discontinuation of a successful treatment will result in major hair loss in a rapid fashion to the level genetically programmed at the time of medication cessation. Oral anti-androgenic medication (finasteride) can be used by some patients, but its use has potential side effects, ranging from sexual dysfunction to high-grade prostate cancer [18]. Topical application of finasteride has shown some efficacy in some clinical studies [18]. Surgically, hair transplantation can be helpful for patients to move hair from a scalp area with normal hair to a location with alopecia, but there is no net gain of total hair as a result of the procedure; it is simply a method of hair redistribution from a normally haired location to a bald area [19].

For patients affected by autoimmunity-mediated alopecia areata, which affects 0.1% to 0.2% population, the current main treatment options are corticosteroids [8, 10]. In cases of small patches of alopecia areata, intra-lesional injections of corticosteroid are commonly utilized, typically performed at a monthly interval [8]. However, for those patients suffering from a more widespread form of autoimmune alopecia (alopecia totalis and alopecia universalis), intra-lesional administration of corticosteroid is not feasible due to the large areas of involvement. While systemic corticosteroid may provide a short-term solution for these patients affected by generalized autoimmune alopecia, long-term treatment of systemic corticosteroid would not be in the best interest of the patients, considering the serious steroid-induced side effects, such as cataracts, hypertension, hyperglycemia/diabetes, osteoporosis/bone fracture, GI bleeding, myocardial infarction, and immunosuppression. In addition, there are substantial economic costs for the patients who receive the medication and their families [20]. Alternatively, systemic immunosuppression (such as mycophenolate mofetil) is an option, but the potential side effects, such as opportunistic infections, progressive multifocal leukoencephalopathy, malignancy, and chronic enteropathy, could be serious with long-term use, and relapse will likely to occur once the immunosuppressive treatment is stopped [21, 22]. In all forms of therapies, the failure rates are high [8].

As mentioned earlier, there is currently no effective medical treatment to reverse hair loss in scarring forms of alopecia since the hair follicles in the scarred scalps of these patients have been permanently destroyed and replaced by fibrous tissues as a result of the underlying inflammatory processes. Medical treatments can be offered to these patients only for the purpose of preventing further, inflammation-induced hair loss, but not for restoring the lost hair. In general, the medical treatments to prevent further scarring in these patients do not typically produce a successful outcome [10].

Thus, for the reasons mentioned here, better hair restoration treatment options are needed. Bioprinted hair follicles, if able to provide a way to restore loss hair, would be a great benefit to patients suffering from a variety of forms of alopecia.

THE TECHNOLOGY: MAKING THE HUMAN HAIR FOLLICLE CONSTRUCT

Having delineated the need for bioengineered hair, the details of the making of a human hair follicle construct will be depicted in the paragraphs that follow to ensure the primary users, our physicians, have a complete understanding, which will naturally lead to their confidence in using the products [23]. Engineering a hair follicle is a huge undertaking. It requires not only that the appropriate cells are included in the bioink (bioprinting materials), but also the understanding of the molecular mechanisms underlying the formation of hair follicle, hair growth, and cycling, as we need to turn cells in a fluid medium into a solid, unique, 3-D longitudinal, round, column-like structure and to ensure the hair growth potential of the finished construct.

Key Steps of Understanding

Before their successful construction of bioprinted hair follicles, these researchers first delineated a few key processes that were critical to the formation of functional hair follicles. First, they gained the knowledge that a kind of specialized mesenchymal cell, termed the dermal papilla cell, is essential for the morphogenesis and cycling of hair follicles. Furthermore, they came to the understanding that the interactions between the epidermal component and the mesenchymal component and the interaction between the cell and the matrix are essential for hair follicle morphogenesis [24]. In addition, utilizing a systems biology approach, these researchers were able to identify and characterize several master regulator genes they could utilize to restore the hair inductive transcriptional signature of the dermal papilla cells. Moreover, they discovered that vasculature is also critical for the in-tissue survival of the engrafted bioprinted constructs.

Construction of the Dermis Formation

The bioprinting process was a laser-based, nozzle-free method, and it was carried out using an Objet24 3-D printer equipped with six well-plate transwell inserts and a UV-curing material VeroWhite (obtained from Stratasys, Los Angeles, California). The researchers utilized microfabricated plastic molds containing hair follicle–shaped extensions, which are adjustable in length, diameter, and density to perform 3-D printing, in order to control the spatial arrangement of the cells in the hair constructs. The bioink for the dermis base contains collagen gel and human foreskin–derived dermal fibroblasts (4 mL of 1.25×10^5/mL fibroblasts in type I collagen matrix). After polymerization of the dermal component at 37°C for 30 minutes, the subsequent seeding of dermal papilla cells (3,000 cells in 100 micro liter per microwell, isolated from adult scalp tissues) over these microwells, the dermal construct was cultured in DMEM with 10% fetal bovine serum at 37°C overnight (total 7 million dermal papilla cells per mL for 255 hair follicles per cm²). This process resulted in formation of aggregate at the base of these wells. By adjusting the diameter of these microwells, these researchers were able to precisely control the aggregated dermal papilla cells size. Furthermore, these aggregations restored the versican (VCAN) and alkaline phosphatase activities but suppressed smooth muscle actin (SMA) expression. VCAN, a large chondroitin sulfate proteoglycan, is a marker of dermal papilla cells and hair growth potential, and its expression is substantially reduced in the dermal papilla of aging hair follicles compared to that of young adult hair follicles [24, 25]. In situ hybridization and immunohistology studies revealed that the mRNA and protein expressions of VCAN were strong in the dermal papilla of anagen (actively growing) hair follicles and were greatly reduced in the dermal papilla of catagen (involution, growth termination, regression) and telogen (resting, quiescence) hair follicles [26]. This hair cycle–specific expression pattern suggests the role of VCAN in the induction of hair morphogenesis, the initiation of hair regeneration, and the maintenance of normal hair growth [27].

Epithelialization

Following the dermal construction, these researchers then moved to induce the differentiation process of the hair follicle by seeding human foreskin-derived keratinocytes over the dermal construct. Keratinocytes (1 million, in DMEM with 10% fetal bovine serum) were allowed to settle down and fill up the microwells and were incubated in a low-calcium epidermalization medium composed of the following (in 500 mL quantity): 75 mL 5 ×

DMEM (Dulbecco's Modified Eagle's Medium), 9.75 mL NaHCO$_3$, 25 mL 5 × Ham's F12 (nutrient mixture), 10 mL L-glutamine, 0.4 mL hydrocortisone, 1 mL ITT, 1 mL EOP, 1 mL adenine, 1 mL selenium, 0.5 mL gentamycin, 1 mL CaCl$_2$, 1.5 mL FCS (fetal calf serum), 1 mL progesterone, and 380 mL sterile milli-Q water in pH 7.0–7.2 [28]. After being cultured for one to three weeks, these epidermal cells engulfed the dermal papilla cell aggregates, forming overlying of keratinocytes, which mimicked hair follicle–like units. Post-addition of keratinocytes, the activities of alkaline phosphatase were found to be sustained in the dermal papilla cells at the base of hair follicle units. Continuous culture of the 3-D printed skin constructs for one week led to differentiation of keratinocytes into lineages in specific hair forms: keratin 5 (marker of the outer root sheath), AE13, AE15, Keratin 71 (markers of the inner root sheath), and keratin 75 (marker of hair medulla and companion layer). Further culturing the 3-D printed skin constructs for three weeks resulted in elongation of the hair follicles down to the dermis, more organization of the inner and outer root sheath layers, and spontaneous repositioning of hair follicle orientation from 90 degrees to an obtuse angle of greater than 120 degrees, resembling the physiological angle observed in human skin. Some hair fibers started to surface as well, suggesting the early success of hair growth even in an *ex vivo* condition.

Genetic Reprogramming

To increase the efficiency of hair follicle induction in the 3-D printed skin constructs, the researchers made use of their prior knowledge of the master regulatory genes critical for dermal papilla cell hair inductive signature. Specifically, they found that overexpression of one of these master regulatory gene, *Lef*-1 (lymphoid enhancer-binding factor 1), could lead to substantial increase in specific hair lineage gene expressions, including keratin 17, keratin 71, keratin 25, and keratin 75. The researchers performed the following transfection. The dermal papilla cells grown into third passage were seeded in six well plates at a density of 100,000 cells per well and cultured overnight. The transfection was then conducted overnight with plasmids pBABE-puro *Lef*-1 (#27023, obtained from Addgene, Cambridge, Massachusetts) and pCMV3-FLI1 (HG14507-UT, obtained from Sino Biological, Beijing, China) in Lipofectamine P3000 transfection reagent (ThermoFisher Scientific, 250 micro liter of reagent with 2.5 micro gram of DNA). Accordingly, overexpression of *Lef*-1 in dermal papilla cells greatly enhanced the success rate of hair follicle induction markers from 19% to 70%.

Vascularization of Hair Follicles

After they learned that 3-D printed skin constructs without vascularization resulted in necrosis and inability for hair growth *in vivo*, these researchers moved forward to conduct vascularization. They co-cultured the skin constructs in the presence of cell medium containing human umbilical vein endothelial cells (2 million cells/ml, obtained from Angio-Proteomie, Boston, Massachusetts) and dermal fibroblasts at a ratio of 16:1 in endothelial cell growth medium (EGM, Angio-Proteomie) supplemented with growth factor (obtained from Lonza, Portsmouth, New Hampshire) for three days. This process resulted in spontaneous capillary formation in the dermis of the constructs, in close proximity to the hair follicles. The subsequent experiments of grafting the vascularized 3-D printed skin constructs onto immunodeficient mice revealed host vascularization into the grafts, confirmed by the immunolabeling of some vessels within the grafts by GS-IB4 (Griffonia simplicifolia isolectin B4, a mouse vascular marker, obtained from ThermoFisher Scientific). In addition, new human vessel lumen formation was observed.

In Vivo Studies

To confirm the true clinical utility of the engineered hair follicles, the researchers engrafted these bioprinted hair follicles onto immunodeficient athymic nude mice (Charles River, Wilmington, Massachusetts) at a high concentration of 255 hair follicles per cm^2 area, in order to be consistent with the density of hair follicles in the human scalp. The engrafting process was preceded by culturing the engineered constructs for one day with 1:1 mixture of two media: EGM-2 and epidermalization medium. A piece of skin (0.8 cm^2) was first removed from the dorsal antero-posterior midline surface of the mice before the placement of the engineered construct into an inserted silicone chamber (1 cm diameter, 1 cm height). Epidermalization medium was added daily to the chamber for five days, and then the chamber was removed, and the engineered construct was sutured onto the mice and secured with bandage for the remaining time of engrafting. After four to five weeks of grafting, substantial hair growth was observed in these grafts; four out of seven mice receiving the grafts had human hair generated successfully. Immunohistology examinations revealed that these successfully engrafted hair follicles did contain differentiated human keratinocytes (as indicated by immunolabeling with K71) and human dermal papilla cells (as confirmed by immunolabeling with VCAN). Interestingly, the absence of the dermal sheath (as evident by the negative immunolabeling with SMAα) did not prevent hair growth, indicating that the combination of keratinocytes and dermal papilla cells is sufficient to generate *de novo* growth of hair follicles. On bright-field microscopic examination, the engineered hair fibers were morphologically similar to those of human terminal hair and possessed an intermediate thickness between human terminal and vellus hair. To ensure that the hair grown in the engrafted areas is of human origin, mRNA extracted from laser-capture microdissection was examined by RT-PCR with a human-specific primer pair, and the process indeed confirmed their human origin.

Conclusions of This Study

The researchers concluded that their biomimetic approach to engineering a human hair follicle skin construct, a bioengineering breakthrough, could soon pave a path for regenerative medicine for skin repair in general and for hair restoration in particular. Figure 5.1 depicts the scheme of the process of making bioprinted human hair follicle.

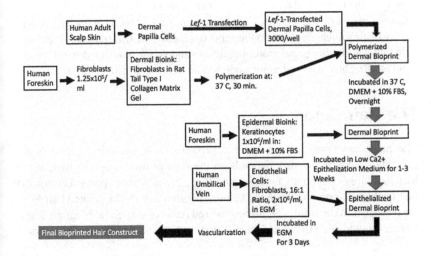

FIGURE 5.1 An operation process for producing bioprinted human hair follicle. (DMEM = Dulbecco's Modified Eagle's Medium; FBS = fetal bovine serum; EGM = endothelial growth medium, *Lef*-1 = master regulatory gene, abbreviation for lymphoid enhancer-binding factor 1.)

UNFINISHED BUSINESS

This section has provided the details of the successful making of a human hair follicle construct. This is a great news for patients affected by alopecia. However, more work needs to be done before it can become a successful commercial product to help patients with hair restoration.

Patient Selection

To successfully utilize the bioprinted hair follicle constructs for the purpose of hair restoration, appropriate patient selection is also a key. Providing a viable hair follicle construct by itself is not sufficient. The other key factor to consider is the host environment. For example, if these engineered hair follicles are to be used for patients suffering from scarring alopecia, do we need to know if the scarred scalps of the recipients have the appropriate matrix milieu and vasculature to accept the construct and sustain the hair growth successfully? For those patients affected by androgenetic alopecia, is there a need for anti-androgenic therapies in parallel with the engrafting of engineered hair follicles for the long-term sustaining of the bioprinted hair follicles? With regard to the patients affected with autoimmune-mediated alopecia, how do we ensure that the immune reaction to the host hair follicle does not do the same damage to the transplanted bioprinted hair follicles? Is this population of patients suitable for bioprinted hair engraftment at all? Thus, we need more studies to answer these critical questions.

The Hair Color

The published paper, so far, has not yet settled on the hair pigment equation. Hair pigment, in turn, depends on the type of melanocyte present at the hair bulb area of the hair follicle [29]. Thus, melanocytes appropriate for the intended hair color would need to be incorporated into the bioprinted hair follicle construct in the future. Semi-customized hair-color-specific bioprinted hair follicles would need to be made available to patients with diverse hair colors.

The Adnexal Structures (Appendages)

Hair follicles situated in the dermal matrix are surrounded by many adnexal structures, and the interaction of hair follicles with these structures may have a role in the sustaining of hair follicles. One such structure is the arrector pili muscle, which attaches to the bulge area of the hair follicle with its known function of contracting the hair (or making goosebumps) in responding to cold temperature or certain emotional states. Recently, studies have pointed out their possible role in maintaining the integrity and stability of hair follicles, and thus their presence in "bioprinted" hair follicles would be another important consideration [30]. In fact, this arrector muscle, together with hair follicles and the sebaceous gland, forms a dermal structure known as a pilosebaceous unit. One piece of indirect evidence in support of the pro–hair stability function of this arrector pili muscle is its absence of attachment to the vellus hair follicle in androgenetic alopecia. The sebaceous gland itself also contributes to the integrity of the hair follicle by providing an oily substance to prevent hair from drying out, and the arrector pili muscle is thought to be involved in this secretion process [30].

The Possibility of Immune Rejection

When the human body receives a foreign implant, whether it is a transplanted heart, a transplanted kidney, or transplanted hair, the immune system is alerted and can mount an antagonistic effort to reject the graft, simply because our immune system is designed this way to fend off invading pathogens, and these implants could be recognized as invaders by our immune cells. Hair follicles are recognized as a site of "immune privilege" [31]. We would need to examine whether the transplanted "bioprinted" hair could break this privilege, leading to autoimmune rejection just like that occurring in alopecia areata [8]. This possibility of immune rejection is especially difficult to deal with when it comes to alopecia areata, which itself is an autoimmune disease that targets hair follicles.

SUMMARY

This chapter delineates a big step forward in hair regenerating medicine. Human hair follicles can now be generated in a laboratory setting, with the ability to regrow lost hair on an animal model. Pending additional issues to be resolved, this regenerated hair follicle could be of great benefit to patients suffering from a variety forms of hair loss.

REFERENCES

1. [3D PRINTING] 3D Printing. Definition of 3D printing. Merriam-Webster. [www.merriam-webster.com/dictionary/3D%20printing] Accessed April 27, 2020.
2. Kacarevic ZP, Rider PM, Alkildani S, et al. An introduction to 3D bioprinting: Possibilities, challenges and future aspects. *Materials (Basel)* 2018; 11(11): 2199. Doi: 10.2290/ma11112199.
3. Chan LS and Srivastava SS. Invention and Innovation. In: Chan LS and Tang WC. Eds. *Engineering-Medicine: Principles and Applications of Engineering in Medicine.* CRC Press, Boca Raton, FL, 2019; pp. 51–65.
4. Schooley S. SWOT analysis: What it is and when to use it. *Business News Daily.* June 23, 2019.
5. Marks DH, Penzi LR, Ibler E, et al. The medical and psychosocial associations of alopecia: Recognizing hair loss as more than a cosmetic concern. *Am J Clin Dermatol* 2019; 20(2): 195–200. Doi: 10.1007/s40257-018-0405-2.
6. Varothai S and Bergfeld WF. Androgenetic alopecia: An evidence-based treatment update. *Am J Clin Dermatol* 2014; 15(3): 217–230. Doi: 10.1007/s40257-014-0077-5.
7. Gupta S, Goyal I, and Mahendra A. Quality of life assessment in patients with androgenetic alopecia. *Int J Trichology* 2019; 11(4): 147–152. Doi: 10.4103/ijt.ijt_6_19.
8. Pratt, CH, King LE, Messenger AG, et al. Alopecia areata. *Nat Rev Dis Primers* 2017; 3: 17011. doi. 10.1038/nrdp.2017.11.
9. Jedlickova H, Niedermeier A, Zgazarovd S, et al. Brunsting-Perry pemphigoid of the scalp with antibodies against laminin 332. *Dermatology* 2011; 222: 193–195. Doi: 10.1159/000322842.
10. Filbrandt R, Rufaut N, Jones L, et al. Primary cicatricial alopecia: Diagnosis and treatment. *CMAJ* 2013; 185(18): 1579–1585. Doi: 10.1503/cmaj.111570.
11. Villasante Fricke AC and Miteva M. Epidemiology and burden of alopecia areata: A systematic review. *Clin Cosmet Investig Dermatol* 2015; 8: 397–403. Doi: 10.2147/CCID.S53985.
12. Safavi KH, Muller SA, Suman VJ, Moshell AN, Melton LJ., 3rd. Incidence of alopecia areata in Olmsted County, Minnesota, 1975 through 1989. *Mayo Clin Proc* 1995; 70(7): 628–633.
13. McMichael AJ, Pearce DJ, Wasserman D, et al. Alpecia in the United States: Outpatient utilization and common prescribing patterns. *J Am Acad Dermatol* 2007; 57(2 suppl): S49–51.
14. Mirzoyev SA, Schrum AG, Davis MD, Torgerson RR. Lifetime incidence risk of alopecia areata estimated at 2.1% by Rochester epidemiology project, 1990–2009. *J Invest Dermatol* 2014; 134: 1141–1142.
15. Russo PM, Fino E, Mancini C, Mazzetti M, Starace M, Piraccini BM. HrQoL in hair loss-affected patients with alopecia areta, androgenetic alopecia and telogen effluvium: The role of personality traits and psychosocial anxiety. *J Eur Acad Dermatol Venereol* 2019; 33(3): 608–611. Doi: 10.1111/jdv.15327.

16. [SALON IRIS] Quotes to inspire: The best hair quotes for hairdressers. [www.saloniris.com/quotes-about-hair/] Accessed May 20, 2020.
17. Olsen EA, Whiting D, Bergfeld W, et al. A multicenter, randomized, placebo-controlled, double-blind clinical trial of a novel formulation of 5% minoxidil topical foam versus placebo in the treatment of androgenetic alopecia in men. *J Am Acad Dermatol* 2007; 57(5): 767–774. Doi: 10.1016/j.jaad.2007.04.012.
18. Lee SW, Juhasz M, Mobasher P, et al. A systemic review of topical finasteride in the treatment of androgenetic alopecia in men and women. *J Drugs Dermatol* 2018; 17(4): 457–463.
19. Lam SM. *Hair Transplant 360: Advances, Techniques, Business Development, and Global Perspectives.* 1st Ed. Jaypee Hights Medical Publishing, New Delhi, India, 2014.
20. Rice JB, White AG, Scarpati LM, et al. Long-term systemic corticosteroid exposure: A systematic literature review. *Clin Ther* 2017; 39(11): 2216–2229. Doi: 10.1016/j.clinthera.2017.09.011.
21. Orvis AK, Wesson SK, Breza TS, et al. Mycophenolate mofetil in dermatology. *J Am Acad Dermatol* 2009; 60(2): 183–199. Doi: 10.1016/j.jaad.08.049.
22. Marietta EV, Cartee A, Rishi A, et al. Drug-induced enteropathy. *Dig Dis* 2015; 33(2): 215–220. Doi: 10.1159/000370205.
23. Abaci, HE, Coffman A, Doucet Y, et al. Tissue engineering of human hair follicles using a biomimetic developmental approach. *Nature Communication* 2018; 9: 5301. Doi: 10.1038/s41467-018-07579-y.
24. Kishimoto J, Ehama R, Wu L, et al. Selective activation of the versican promoter by epithelial-mesenchymal interactions during hair follicle development. *Proc Natel Acad Sci USA* 1999; 96(13): 7336–7341. Doi: 10.1073/pnas.96.13.7336.
25. Jo SJ, Kim JY, Jang S, et al. Decrease of versican levels in the follicular dermal papilla is a remarkable aging-associated change of human hair follicles. *J Dermatol Sci* 2016; 84(3): 354–357. Doi: 10.1016/j.jdermsci.2016.09.014.
26. Oh JW, Kloepper J, Langan EA, et al. A guide to studying human hair follicle cycle in vivo. *J Invest Dermatol* 2016; 136(1): 34–44. Doi: 10.1038/JID.2015.354.
27. Soma T, Tajima M, and Kishimoto J. Hair cycle-specific expression of versican in human hair follicles. *J Dermatol Sci* 2005; 39: 147–154. Doi: 10.1016/j.jdermsci.2005.03.010.
28. Gangatirkar P, Paquet-Fifield S, Li A, et al. Establishment of 3D organotypic cultures using human neonatal epidermal cells. *Nat. Protoc* 2007; 2: 178–186. Doi: 10.1038/nprot.2006.448.
29. Lin JY and Fisher DE. Melanocyte biology and skin pigmentation. *Nature* 2007; 445: 843–850. https://doi.org/10.1038/nature05660.
30. Torkamani N, Rufaut NW, Jones L, et al. Beyond goosebumps: Does the arrector pili muscle have a role in hair loss? *Int J Trichology* 2014; 6(3): 88–94. Doi: 10.4103/0974-7753.139077.
31. Ito T, Ito N, Bettermann A, et al. Collapse and restoration of MHC class-I-dependent privilege exploiting the human hair follicle as a model. *Am J Pathol* 2004; 164(2): 623–634. Doi: 10.1016/S0002-9440(10)63151-3.

Regeneration of Full-Thickness Human Skin by 3-D Bioprinting

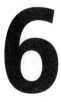

Lawrence S. Chan

Contents

DOI: 10.1201/9781003121275-8

INTRODUCTION

The definition and technical details of 3-D bioprinting were introduced in the chapter prior to this. Briefly, 3-D bioprinting is a manufacturing process in which a functional and biological compatible tissue construct can be produced for the purpose of restoring normal biological functions. Authors of one scholarly publication stated it this way: "Known as 3-D bioprinting, this technology involves the precise layering of cells, biologic scaffolds, and growth factors with the goal of creating bioidentical tissue for a variety of uses" [1]. In this chapter, we will focus on the manufacturing of human skin equivalent.

Although sometimes its importance is taken for granted, skin is actually very important for human survival. Being the biggest organ of the human body, skin serves a critical barrier function [2, 3]. The first function of the skin is to provide a physical barrier to keep the desirable contents inside the body and to keep the undesirable contents outside the body. Every hour, our body is being challenged by undesirable components we encounter, like pathogenic microorganism, irritants, and allergens. An excellent clinical example illustrating this point is a skin barrier protein defect in patients with a mutation of a gene encoding filaggrin, allowing easy entry of undesirable content into the skin. The unfortunate result of filaggrin mutation could lead to a chronic skin inflammation condition commonly known as atopic dermatitis [2]. Furthermore, it is important for the body not only to keep undesirable contents out, but also to keep desirable contents in, such as water and electrolytes. The loss of skin endangers life due to the loss of water and electrolytes in addition to the threat of infection. One such example is the deletion of just a single gene encoding claudin-1, an epidermal tight junctional protein essential for water content preservation, which led to the early demise of animals from severe dehydration secondary to significant trans-epidermal water loss [4]. Another essential but often neglected skin function as a physical barrier is the task of thermoregulation. When our bodies encounter high temperature derived from an external or internal source, skin takes up its role in reducing the excessive heat by increasing sweat. An excellent clinical example is demonstrated in a skin disease called anhidrotic ectodermal dysplasia, in which patients have genetic defects in the development of teeth, sweat glands, and hair, resulting in their inability to sweat or properly regulate temperature [5, 6]. Moreover, skin has a valuable social function, as stated by the Italian artist Michelangelo: "What spirit is so empty and blind, that it cannot recognize the fact that the foot is more noble than the shoe, and skin more beautiful than the garment with which it is clothed?" [7].

The other essential function of the skin is to provide immunological defense for the human. Human skin contains symbiotic bacterial species that defend against pathogenic bacteria. The diminished presence of these "friendly bugs" is linked to increased colonization of pathogenic bacteria and chronic inflammatory skin disease [2]. In addition, human skin possesses antimicrobial peptides such as beta-defensins and cathelicidin, which possess strong antimicrobial properties. Reduction of these peptides is associated with serious, even life-threatening infection events [2]. Moreover, human skin has the presence of immune cells such as antigen-presenting cells and T cells, which survey the skin environment, ready to counter invaders [3]. In the following sections, the rationale (the need) for the production of engineered skin equivalent will be discussed first, followed by a detailed description of the bioprinting of a human skin equivalent. Note that the word "equivalent" will be used interchangeably with substitute, graft, product, or construct.

ANALYSIS OF THE NEED

Having delineated the essential protective functions of skin, we now examine the rationale for manufacturing human skin construct.

Covering for Acute Burn Patients

Skin burns, a major medical emergency, can occur when patients encounter a house fire, electrical currents, caustic chemicals, radiation, automobile accidents, and work-related accidents, and burns can result in major skin loss [8]. Large areas of skin loss can also occur in certain medical conditions, such as skin reaction to medications or infections, resulting in extremely dangerous conditions similar to burns, such as in toxic epidermal necrolysis. In fact, patients suffering from toxic epidermal necrolysis are routinely transferred to burn units for treatment [9, 10]. According to statistics collected by the American Burn Association, 400,000 patients are hospitalized annually for burn injury–related causes, with 300,000 treated at one of the 128 burn centers in the US [11]. When these medical emergencies present in the emergency rooms of hospitals, one of the key factors in saving the affected patients is temporary covering their skin-loss areas, since a large area of open wound would result in substantial water loss, electrolyte depletion, hypothermia, and serious infection [8]. Bioengineered skin constructs have the ability to provide temporary or even permanent skin covering, thus increasing the patients' survival and quality of life [12].

Healing Materials for Chronic Wounds

Chronic wound healing is a significant medical issue, especially for the elderly population, and chronic wounds impose substantial morbidity and mortality on a large number of older patients [13]. According to statistics collected by the Wound Healing Society, about 6.5 million people in the US are affected by chronic wounds, and the inability of normal healing of wound, scars, and adhesions poses a major health problem in the US and worldwide. The problem is especially prominent in the aging population, among whom several diseases that can exacerbate wound healing problems, such as diabetes, chronic venous insufficiency, and atherosclerosis, are highly prevalent [13, 14]. Chronic wound care costs about $10 billion in the US annually. Since cellular products containing keratinocytes, fibroblasts, and fibrin matrix in a fluid form have been shown to substantially promote wound healing, engineered skin tissue composed of these cellular products in a solid form would potentially provide even better healing benefits [13].

Viable Models for Skin Disease Investigation

Because of the inherent limitation and ethical concern with regard to the use of live animals as skin disease models, bioengineered skin is being considered as a potential substitute for skin disease modeling [15, 16]. A 3-D fully humanized skin equivalent, comprising a stratified and terminally differentiated epidermis and a dermal compartment consisting of fibroblast-generated extracellular matrix has been shown to be a good model for studying melanoma invasion [17]. The available 3-D bioprinted skin construct containing vasculature, in addition to epidermis and fibroblast matrix, would provide an even better and more natural modeling material for the study of diseases. Particularly useful models are those for cancer mechanism study [18].

Platform for Drug-Delivery Studies

Recent advances in biotechnology enable the generation of full-thickness skin constructs resembling complex human skin structure with appendages, vasculatures, nerves, hair follicles, pigmented and immune cells, and hypodermis. Such bioengineered skin constructs can enhance the ability of pharmaceutical companies to test drug delivery at the early stage of studies in a time-saving and resource-savvy manner. In addition, fewer animals are needed to conduct these drug-delivery studies [15, 16, 18].

THE TECHNOLOGY: MAKING 3-D BIOPRINTED SKIN

Two major methods of bioengineering skin constructs are electrospinning and 3-D bioprinting [19]. In the following paragraphs, the detailed processes of making 3-D bioprinted full-thickness human skin containing a vascularized and perfusable dermis will be discussed, based on a recent paper published in 2020 [20].

Vascularized and Perfusable Skin Grafts: Rationale and Cellular Components

In the past, skin graft construction has provided temporary coverage for wounds. Skin grafts that can only provide temporary coverage, although helping prevent skin infection, do not provide a solution to the healing of chronic wounds. The major disadvantage of temporary coverage is that patients with a chronic wound-healing problem cannot complete epithelialization in the areas of the wound due to a variety of underlying medical conditions, notably aging-related healing inability, cardiovascular insufficiency, and diabetes. Apligraf, one of the currently available skin graft products, suffers from this disadvantage, likely due to its lack of dermal vascularization. In order to construct a skin graft that can be permanently incorporated into the skin, researchers have looked into methods that can accomplish that goal. Toward this end, a group of medical researchers tried to perform 3-D bioprinting of a skin graft consisting of four live human skin cells: keratinocytes, fibroblasts, endothelial cells, and pericytes. While endothelial cells function to form the inner lining of vasculature, pericytes are functionally situated on the outer surface of vasculature. Located at the precapillary arteriole, capillary, and postcapillary venule, pericytes, which are labeled by antibody to growth factor receptor PDGFRβ and proteoglycan NG2 (a co-receptor of PDGF), are known to have contractile ability and a blood flow–controlling function [21]. These researchers have indeed achieved this important goal of successful printing a vascularized skin substitute [20]. The following paragraphs detail the equipment, biomaterials, and bioprinting process used by this group of researchers and the confirmation *in vitro* and *in vivo* studies of this engineered skin product will be described and discussed.

The Bioprinting Process

The bioprinting was performed with a commercially available Bio X bioprinter (obtained from CELLINK Life Sciences, Brighton, UK) with the following technical specifications: sterile 30-gauge stainless steel blunt needle. The process is divided into two parts. In the first "bioink" layer, three types of human cells—fibroblasts, pericytes, and endothelial cells—were mixed with and suspended in a rat tail type I collagen milieu. The fibroblasts were derived from human foreskin, the pericytes were derived from placenta, and the endothelial cells were derived from umbilical cord blood endothelial cell colony-forming cells. During the early stage of their study, these researchers learned that the ratio of pericytes to the other cell types significantly influenced the collagen contraction. After *in vitro* experiments that predetermined an optimal ratio of these three cell types without causing collagen contraction, the final "bioink" was formulated with 7×10^5/mL fibroblasts, 7×10^5/mL endothelial cells, and 3.5×10^5/mL pericytes, suspended in a solution composed of 2.2 mL of 3.5 mg/mL rat tail type I collagen (obtained from Corning, Glendale, Arizona), 150 micro liters of fetal bovine serum (obtained from R & D Systems, Minneapolis, Minnesota), 290 micro liters of 10X pH reconstitution buffer (0.05 M NaOH, 2.2% $NaHCO_3$, and 200 mM HEPES), and 290 micro liters of 10X HAMP-F12 medium (obtained from Gibco/Thermo Fisher Scientific, Waltham, Massachusetts) and kept at 4°C to prevent gelation. The bioprinting of this first layer forms the bioprinted "dermis" with these specific parameters: 2.9 mL of dermal bioink, at a resolution of 300 micro meters; 6 psi pneumatic pressure, placed on top of a six-well Transwell PET insert with 3 micro meter pore size. The dermal component of the bioprint was conducted at 4°C, at extrusion pressure of 50 kPa for 205 seconds. After the completion of the dermal bioprint, the constructs were incubated in EGM2 medium (obtained from Lonza, Portsmouth, New Hampshire) for four days to allow self-assembly of endothelial networks. Note that these researchers found that EGM2 medium was essential in the endothelial network assembly.

Following the first "bioink" layer, the second "bioink" layer, formulated to contain human foreskin–derived keratinocytes (2×10^6/mL) in 500 micro liters of 1:1 keratinocyte growth medium (obtained from Lonza) and skin differentiation medium were utilized to bioprint to form the "epidermal" layer with these specific parameters: 500 micro liters of bioink, 300 micro meter resolution, 2.5 psi pneumatic pressure, placed on top of the 3-D dermal construct. The composition of the skin differentiation medium is: DEM/HAM's F-12 (3:1), supplemented with 10% fetal bovine serum, 0.1nM cholear toxin (obtained from Sigma, St. Louis, Missouri), 0.4 µg/mL hydrocortisone-21 (Sigma), 5 µg/mL insulin (Sigma), 5 µg/mL apotransferrin (Sigma), and 0.5 ng/mL epidermal growth factor (obtained from Peprotech, Cranbury, New Jersey). The epidermal part of the bioprint was achieved (at day four) with a sterile 32-gauge stainless steel blunt needle at extrusion pressure of 35 kPa for 54 seconds.

Post-Printing Processing

After the printing process was completed for the "dermal" and "epidermal" layers, 1 mL of acellular epidermal bioink milieu (without keratinocytes) was added to the bottom compartment of the six-well Transwell insert and incubated for 24 hours at 37°C. Then the media were removed and replaced by 100% skin differentiation medium (described earlier) for four days, before placing the bioprinted product onto the immunodeficient mice for *in vivo* study.

Figure 6.1 depicts the process for bioprinting skin.

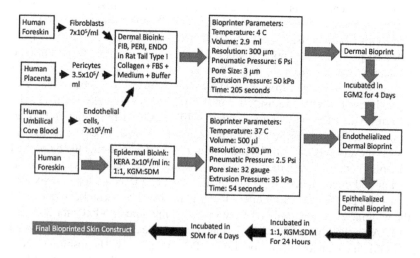

FIGURE 6.1 The flow of operation process for bioprinting skin. (FIB = fibroblasts; PERI = pericytes; ENDO = endothelial cells; KERA = keratinocytes; FBS = fetal bovine serum; KGM = keratinocyte growth medium; SDM = skin differentiation medium; EGM = endothelial growth medium.

Morphology Confirmation by *In Vitro* Studies

The bioprinted skin products were cultured at air-liquid interface starting at day 4 to foster tissue maturation. Histology and immunohistology examinations at day 30 showed substantial maturation of fibroblast distribution in the "dermis" (the first "bioink" layer) and keratinocyte organization in the "epidermis" compartments (the second "bioink" layer). The "epidermis" layer showed the formation of multilayers of keratinocytes, organizing into an "epidermal" barrier by evidence of the presence of filaggrin (a marker of stratum corneum layer), cytokeratin 14 (a marker of basal cell layer), cytokeratin 10 (a marker of superbasal layers), and type IV collagen (a marker of skin basement membrane). Another observation of epidermal maturation was the well-organized cuboidal basal cells adherent to the basement membrane. Within the dermal side of the bioprint, endothelial cells and pericytes organized to form interconnected microvascular networks. As early as day 10 post printing, the presence of human CD31+ (a marker of endothelial cells) vessel-like structures were observed in the "dermis" compartment.

Structural and Functional Confirmation by *In Vivo* Studies

To examine the biological compatibility of the bioprinted product, skin grafts were placed on the backs of immunodeficient mice to test its ability to incorporate into the skin of the recipient host. After small pieces of skin were removed from the dorsal side of the mice, a comparable size of bioprinted skin products were sutured onto the mice under sterile operating conditions. At two weeks post engrafting, vascular structures were formed (as demonstrated by UEA-1, Ulex Europaeus agglutinin 1, staining), and epidermal maturation was evident by the expressions of cytokeratins 10 and 14 on the grafts. At four weeks post engrafting, immunohistology demonstrated the presence of vessel formation (by human CD31+ staining), host microvascular infiltration (by staining of GSL-B4+, a marker of mouse endothelial cells), and epidermal maturation (by human involucrin+ and laminin 5+ staining and rete ridge-like structure formation). Interestingly, the inclusion of pericytes in the dermal "bioink" enhanced the maturation and the thickness of the epidermal layer of the engineered skin grafts, as demonstrated by increased expressions of laminin 5 and cytokeratin 10 and enhanced formation of rete ridge-like skin structure. Moreover, the addition of pericytes to the dermal "bioink" promoted the host microvascular infiltration to the skin graft, as illustrated by the increased expression of GSL-B4.

The microvascular networks formed inside the bioprinted product organized to connect with the host microvasculature, and at four weeks post engrafting, the blood perfusion had established within the microcirculation of the bioprinted skin graft. The assessment of perfusion was conducted as follows: Diluted fluorescein UEA 1 (obtained from Vector Laboratories, Burlingame, California) with normal saline solution was injected into the mice bearing the engineered bioprinted skin through their tail vein. After administering 200 micro liters of the test solution, the mice were euthanized 30 minutes later, allowing the test solution to circulate. The harvested engineered skin grafts were divided in half, with one half fixed in 10% buffered formalin for paraffin embedding (for regular histology examination) and the second half embedded in OCT compound for cryo-sectioning (for immunohistology examinations). The skin sections confirmed the staining of UAE 1 on human endothelial cells in the engineered skin graft, thus indicating the establishment of vascular perfusion within the bioprinted skin.

Conclusion on Bioprinted Skin

These researchers concluded that the 3-D bioprinting method can be utilized to construct, with live human keratinocytes, fibroblasts, endothelial cells, and pericytes, a multilayered and stratified structure of skin equivalent that is vascularized and perfusable. To the best of my knowledge, this report represents the most advanced bioengineered human skin to date [20].

UNFINISHED BUSINESS

While the success of the manufacturing process of 3-D bioprinted human skin is indeed exciting, several important questions remain to be answered.

Physiological Functionality

Some of the natural functions of human skin have so far not been demonstrated in this most recent bioengineered skin construct, such as sensation, UV protection, excretion, perspiration, and thermal regulation [12, 22]. Moreover, engineered skin products will need to provide the proper pigmentation if they are to be useful as a permanent replacement [15]. In addition, the importance of the neuro-immuno-cutaneous system in bioengineered skin design cannot be underestimated, as the skin is an essential sensory organ, and the presence of the neurological component is important for engineered skin to provide so as to fulfill its complete biological functions. Furthermore, proper function of engineered skin also will need a viable lymphatic vessel system, in addition to a perfusable blood vessel system [15, 23, 24]. In addition, the essential presence of functional adnexal structures (appendages), such as sweat glands, sebaceous glands, and hair follicles (and their associated arrector pili muscle), will need to be addressed. Sebaceous glands provide an innate immune defense function against microorganisms as well as a lubricating function for the skin, and hair follicles provide a cosmetic function in addition to a thermoregulatory function, which is also supplied by the sweat glands. Furthermore, the fact that some patients who recently received "bioprinted skin" experienced neurological abnormalities, such as lack of sensation or chronic pain, indicates the need for further research [22, 25]. The recent success of 3-D bioprinting in producing vascularized human hair follicles, which were shown to be functional by their taking root in immunodeficient mice, is a significant step forward for fulfilling the need in this aspect [26].

Skin Color

So far, the published paper has not yet settled the skin pigment equation. Skin pigment, in turn, depends on the type of melanocyte present in the skin [27]. Thus, melanocytes appropriate for the intended skin color would need to be incorporated into the bioprinted skin construct in the future, if the engineered products are to be permanently incorporated into the host skin.

Immunologically Protecting Functions

Since natural skin is not only a physical barrier but also an immunological barrier, providing both innate and acquired immune functions essential in defending the human host against undesirable invaders such as bacteria and fungi, these immune capacities will need to be appropriately provided by the bioengineered skin construct, if these constructs are to provide the full functionality of the natural skin [2, 28]. At a minimum, we will need to study whether the "bioprinted" skin product can provide the needed innate immune defense components: namely, the antimicrobial peptides—human beta defensins and cathelicidin (LL-37). Because beta defensins and LL-37 are products of keratinocytes, these functions are conceivably present in the engineered skin [2, 29]. As for the adaptive immune system, it is possible that the host immune system could eventually deliver the needed T cells and antigen-presenting cells to the "bioprinted" skin graft. In the 2020 article, host macrophages (as marked by F4/80+ labeling), one type of mouse antigen-presenting cells, were detected in the dermal infiltrates of the engineered skin engrafted on the back of the mouse [20]. It is reasonable to assume that T cells from the host could also infiltrate the engrafted skin, thus providing the adaptive immune protection.

Immune Rejection

Unlike fibroblasts, endothelial cells can act as non-professional antigen presenting cells, with the ability to present Class I and Class II HLA antigens to host T cells. In light of this, immune rejection of engineered skin construct is a potential problem. As suggested by the field experts, deleting the ability to present antigens by CRISPR/Cas9-mediated gene editing methodology can provide a way to eliminate the possibility of endothelial cell-mediated immune rejection [20, 30].

Potential Holdup

Since the construction of engineered skin requires lots of live cells, this can become a bottleneck for the applicability of this innovation. The challenges are that only small quantity of cells can be harvested from skin biopsies, and it is unfeasible to harvest these cells from patients with diabetes, severe burns, or chronic wounds. The endothelial cell colony-forming cells available from human umbilical cord blood and adult peripheral blood will provide an excellent source of endothelial cells, since these cells can be expanded to more than 100 population doublings and can also be cloned. The source of pericytes can be obtained from human placenta. The most limited cells come down to keratinocytes and fibroblasts [20].

SUMMARY

The recent success in constructing 3-D bioprinted skin equivalent with the presence of perfusable blood vessels is a great step forward to fulfill the need of bioengineered skin for many medical applications. Some technical challenges remain to be solved before functional bioprinted skin will be routinely available for clinic use as a permanent replacement for lost skin.

REFERENCES

1. Bishop ES, Mostafa S, Pakvasa M, et al. 3-D bioprinting technologies in tissue engineering and regenerative medicine: Current and future trends. *Genes & Diseases* 2017; 4(4): 185–195. https://doi.org/10.1016/j.gendis.2017.10.002.

2. Chan LS. Keratinocytes. In: Chan LS and Shi VY. Eds. *Atopic Dermatitis: Inside Out or Outside In?* Elsevier, New York, NY, 2020a.

3. Nguyen AV and Soulika AM. The dynamics of the skin's immune system. *Int J Mol Sci* 2019; 20(8): 1811. Doi: 10.3390/ijms20081811.

4. Furuse M, Hata M, Furuse K, et al. Claudin-based tight junctions are crucial for the mammalian epidermal barrier: A lesson from claudin-1-deficient mice. *J Cell Biol* 2002; 156(6): 1099–1111. Doi: 10.1083/jcb.200110122.

5. Jones KB, Goodwin AF, Landan M, et al. Characterization of x-linked hypohidrotic ectodermal dysplasia (XL-HED) hair and sweat gland phenotypes using phototichogram analysis and live confocal imaging. *Am J Med Genet* 2013; (7): 1585–1593. Doi: 10.1002/ajmg.a.35959.

6. Timothy W, Fete M, Schneider H, et al. Ectodermal dysplasia: Classification and organization by phenotype, genotype, and molecular pathway. *Am J Med Genet* 2019; 179(3): 442–447. Doi: 10.1002/ajmg.a.61045.

7. [BRAINY QUOTE] [brainyquote.com/quotes/Michelangelo_183582?src=t_skin] Accessed May 25, 2020.

8. Lang TC, Zhao R, Kim A, et al. A critical update of the assessment and acute management of patients with severe burns. *Adv Wound Care* 2019; 8(12): 607–633. Doi: 10.1089/woud.2019.0963.

9. Roujeau JC, Kelly JP, Naldi L, et al. Medication use and the risk of Stevens-Johnson Syndrome or toxic epidermal necrolysis. *N Engl J Med* 1995; 333: 1600–1608. Doi: 10.1016/NEJM199512143332404.

10. Mockenhaupt M. The current understanding of Stevens-Johnson syndrome and toxic epidermal necrolysis. *Expert Rev Clin Immunol* 2011; 7(6): 803–815. https://doi.org/10.1586/eci.11.66.

11. [ABA] Burn incidence fact sheet. American Burn Association. [www.ameriburn.org/who-we-are/media/burn-incidence-fact-sheet/] Accessed May 26, 2020.

12. Shpichka A, Butnaru D, Bezrukov EA, Sukhanov RB, Atala A, Burdukovskii V, Zhang Y, Timashev P. Skin tissue regeneration for burn injury. *Stem Cell Res Ther* 2019; 10: 94. Doi: 10.1186/s13287-019-1203-3.

13. Gould L, Abadir P, Brem H, et al. Chronic wound repair and healing in older adults: Current status and future research. *J Am Geriatr Soc* 2015; 63(3): 427–438. Doi: 10.1111/jgs.13332.

14. [WOUND] Wound healing society. [www.woundheal.org] Accessed May 26, 2020.

15. Abaci HE, Guo Z, Doucet Y, et al. Next generation human skin constructs as advanced tools for drug development. *Exp Biol Med (Maywood)* 2017; 242(17): 1657–1668. Doi: 10.1177/1535370217712690.

16. Sarkiri M, Fox SC, Fratila-Apachitei LE, Zadpoor AA. Bioengineered skin intended for skin disease modeling. *Int J Mol Sci* 2019; 20(6): 1507. Doi: 10.3390/ijms20061407.

17. Hill DS, Robinson NDP, Caley MP, Chen M, O'Toole EA, Armstrong JL, Przyborski S, Lovat PE. A novel fully-humanized 3D skin equivalent to model early melanoma invasion. *Mol Cancer Ther* 2015; 14(11): 2665–2673. Doi: 10.1158/1535-7163.MCT-15-0394.

18. Charbe N, McCarron PA, and Tambuwala MM. Three-dimensional bio-printing: A new frontier in oncology research. *World J Clin Oncol* 2017; 8(1): 21–36. Doi: 10.5306/ajco.v8.i1.21.

19. Randall MJ, Jungel A, Rimann M, Wuertz-Kozak K. Advances in the biofabrication of 3D skin in vitro: Healthy and pathological models. *Front Bioeng Biotechnol* 2018; 6: 154. Doi: 10.3389/fbioe.2018.00154.

20. Baltazar T, Merola J, Catrino C, et al. Three dimensional bioprinting of a vascularized and perfusable skin graft using human keratinocytes, fibroblasts, pericytes, and endothelial cells. *Tissue Engineering: Part A* 2020; 26(5–6): 227–238. Doi: 10.1089/ten.tea.2019.0201.

21. Attwell D, Mishra A, Hall CN, et al. What is a pericyte? *J Cereb Blood Metab* 2016; 36(2): 451–455. Doi: 10.1177/0271678X15610340.

22. Weng T, Wu P, Zhang W, et al. Regeneration of skin appendages and nerves: Current status and further challenges. *J Transl Med* 2020; 18: 53. Doi: 10.1186/s12967-020-02248-5.

23. Chan LS. Microcirculation. In: Chan LS and Shi VY. Eds. *Atopic Dermatitis: Inside Out or Outside In?* Elsevier, New York, NY, 2020b.

24. Vidal Yucha SE, Tamamoto KA, Kaplan DL. The importance of the neuro-immuno-cutaneous system on human skin equivalent design. *Cell Prolif* 2019; 52(6): e12677. Doi: 10.1111/cpr.12677.

25. Torkamani N, Rufaut NW, Jones L, et al. Beyond goosebumps: Does the arrector pili muscle have a role in hair loss? *Int J Trichology* 2014; 6(3): 88–94. Doi: 10.4103/0974-7753.139077.

26. Abaci HE, Coffman A, Doucet Y, et al. Tissue engineering of human hair follicles using a biomimetic developmental approach. *Nat Communication* 2018. Doi: 10.1038/s41467-018-07579-y.

27. Lin JY and Fisher DE. Melanocyte biology and skin pigmentation. *Nature* 2007; 445: 843–850. https://doi.org/10.1038/nature05660.

28. Kobayashi T, Naik S, Nagao K. Choreographing immunity in the skin epithelial barrier. *Immunity* 2019; 50(3): 552–565. Doi: 10.1016/j.immuni.2019.02.023.

29. Schauber J and Gallo RL. Antimicrobial peptides and the skin immune defense system. *J Allergy Clin Immunol* 2008; 122(2): 261–266. Doi: 10.1016/j.jaci.2008.03.027.

30. Chan LS. Precision. In: Chan LS and Tang WC. Eds. *Engineering-Medicine: Principles and Applications of Engineering in Medicine.* CRC Press, Boca Raton, FL, 2019.

Regeneration of Natural Skin Barrier

An Eco-Friendly Approach to Atopic Dermatitis Therapy

Angelina G. Chan

Contents

DOI: 10.1201/9781003121275-9

INTRODUCTION

Regeneration, as depicted in this chapter, describes methods to restore the natural skin barrier defects that are important factors contributing to the pathogenesis of atopic dermatitis (AD). Two major defects of functionally interconnected barriers that need to be restored in the skin of AD patients are physical and immune barriers. Restoring these barriers by topically applied and eco-friendly methods will be the central focus of this chapter.

ANALYSIS OF THE NEED

As a chronic inflammatory skin condition, AD affects about 10% to 20% of children and 1% to 7% of adults. The major symptoms of AD include skin inflammation, itchiness, and related infection [1, 2]. Although not a life-threatening disease, AD does carry a huge disease burden, costing an estimated US $5.3 billion in 2015 [3]. AD is also considered the first step in the atopic march, a process leading to the development of allergic rhinitis or asthma, further contributing to disease burden [4].

The pathogenesis of AD is a multi-factorial process, with key disease development elements including skin barrier defects and immune dysregulation [5–7]. Both physical barrier and immune barrier defects have been documented in AD patients.

Physical Barrier and Its Defect in AD

Skin is the major physical barrier of the human body, with the epidermis as a major component. The normal epidermis is approximately 15 to 30 nm thick and contains cells, cellular proteins, and lipids, with four major layers: stratum corneum, stratum granulosum, stratum spinosum, and stratum basale [5, 8, 9]. These layers are created through keratinization, a process in which keratinocytes are terminally differentiated and progressively migrate from the basal cell layers to the stratum corneum [9].

One main function of the skin is to serve as a physical barrier between an organism's internal and external environments [9]. In the stratum corneum, this barrier is formed by cross-linked epidermal barrier proteins, including filaggrin (filament-aggregating protein, FLG), keratins, thyroglobulin, and loricrin [8]. Below the stratum corneum, barriers include epidermal tight junctions (TJs) and the basement membrane zone [9].

Physical barrier dysfunction is a major pathophysiologic component of AD, including mutations in genes encoding FLG (molecular size 37 kDa), corneodesmosin, as well as related polymorphisms in genes encoding serine peptidase inhibitor Kazal-type 5 (SPINK5) and serine protease kallikrein-related peptidase-7 (KLK7) [9, 10]. Moreover, reduced expression and dysfunction of the lipid and protein of the skin barrier, such as FLG, involucrin, loricrin, and TJ protein claudins induced by overexpression of Th2 and Th22 cytokines, are observed in AD [8, 11]. Null mutations in the FLG gene, especially those that are homozygous, are linked to impairment of the skin barrier and an increased risk of developing AD [6, 9, 12, 13]. Although about 40% to 60% of individuals with the FLG null mutation do not develop the disease of AD, and many who have AD may outgrow the disease, disruption of the expression of the FLG gene is shown to lead to an increased risk of AD [5, 6]. Epigenetic changes, whether inherited or caused by environmental exposures, through DNA methylation or post-transcriptional regulation, could also be a risk [6]. FLG mutations were found to increase the risk of eczema as well as asthma and rhinitis, revealing a link between FLG gene alteration and extra-cutaneous inflammatory diseases [14, 15].

Other major defects in AD skin causing impairment of skin function involve the lipid bilayer and TJs [8, 12]. One study of 27 AD patients found a correlation between abnormal composition of stratum corneum lipids and pathogenic S. aureus colonization. More specifically, the study found that levels of certain ceramides and triglycerides were significantly lower in S. aureus-colonized than S. aureus-non-colonized participants, suggesting a link between pathogen colonization and lipid composition abnormality [16]. TJs are intercellular barriers that can selectively regulate which solutes can pass the epithelium, thus functioning as a second barrier structure [9, 12]. TJs are composed of many proteins, of which claudin-1 and -23 were found to have a reduced expression in AD skin at both the mRNA and the protein levels [17]. Experimentally, claudin-1-deficient mice died with wrinkled skin and dehydration within one day of birth, indicating the critical role of claudin in barrier function [18].

Immune Barrier and Its Defect in AD

Many studies have documented AD's immune dysfunction affecting both the innate and adaptive components [19]. The innate immune defense—namely, commensal bacteria and antimicrobial peptides—will be the focus.

Bacteria and other microorganisms are naturally present in normal human skin. As a complex microbiome, human skin is colonized by many commensal bacteria, which participate in the defense against pathogenic organisms such as *S. aureus* [20]. Coagulase-negative staphylococci (CoNS) are one example of commensal bacteria, with production of antimicrobial molecules against *S. aureus* [20, 21].

Dysbiosis defines a condition in which the composition of resident commensal microorganism communities is altered, relative to the community found in healthy individuals [22]. This often results in loss of microorganism diversity, including many symbiotic bacteria; a disruption of homeostasis; and the predominance of one pathogen [23, 24]. Dysbiosis is linked to the development of many inflammatory skin diseases, including acne, psoriasis, and hidradenitis suppurativa, as well as AD [20, 23–25]. Dysregulation of the skin microbiome is often induced by environmental factors, including temperature, use of antibiotics, pH, infections, hygiene, or dryness, as well as genetic mutations [23–25]. The AD skin microbiome is often characterized by a deficiency in microbiota diversity and colonization by the pathogen *S. aureus* (50%–60% toxin-producing), occurring in approximately 90% of patients with AD [21, 24, 26–28]. *S. aureus* colonization is linked to later development of AD, indicating the importance of the microbiome in the pathogenesis of AD and suggesting that *S. aureus* may, in fact, cause AD [24, 27].

Dysbiosis is also linked to reduced levels of antimicrobial peptides (AMPs) present in AD skin and certain skin conditions such as pH, as *S. aureus* tends to grow better in the more basic skin conditions present in AD patients [20, 21]. This may be tied to defects in FLG proteins. Since the degradation products of FLG protein generate an acidic condition, the reduction of these products promotes *S. aureus* growth. *S. aureus* colonizes AD skin through the formation of biofilms, which enable the bacterial to grow rapidly on the epidermis [21]. Furthermore, various toxins produced by *S. aureus*, like proteases, α-toxin, δ-toxin, enterotoxins, and superantigens, may contribute to inflammation and impairment of skin immune barrier function [24, 28]. During untreated flares of AD, the abundance of *S. aureus* increases, while the abundance of *S. epidermis*—a type of commensal bacteria that can produce antimicrobials (such as AMPs) and thus may limit colonization of *S. aureus*—decreases [21, 24, 29].

Importantly, the severity of the disease in AD patients has been shown to vary with skin microbiome composition: *S. aureus* and *S. epidermis* tend to be more prevalent in patients with more severe AD and in patients with less severe AD, respectively [21, 30].

Antimicrobials, whether synthetic or naturally present, are an essential defense mechanism against various pathogens [31]. Antimicrobial peptides (AMPs), also known as host defense peptides, are one example of a naturally present compound that functions in all organisms to control microbial infections and have been identified in mammals, plants, fungi, amphibians, insects, crustaceans, fish, echinoderms, and bacteria [32]. They are an important part of the first line of defense, especially for eukaryotes such as plants and fungi and invertebrate animals that do not have an adaptive immunity [33]. In mammals, AMPs that have been identified include defensin, LL-37, histatin, lactoferricin, protegrin, and indolicidin [32]. In humans, 20 known AMPs are present in the skin, including human β-defensin-1, 2, 3, and 4; the cathelicidin LL-37; and the dermcidin peptide [19, 34].

With direct antimicrobial properties, AMPs function as a part of organisms' innate immunity [34]. Though AMPs have many different mechanisms of action, the two major methods are immune modulation and direct killing [33]. In terms of immune modulation, AMPs can activate immune responses and recruit immune cells through chemoattraction, including dendritic cells, mast cells, and leukocytes in humans, and can help limit or reduce inflammation. For direct killing, AMPs use the mechanism of membrane targeting through electrostatic charge or hydrophobicity of the membrane lipids, as membrane-targeting AMPs can differentiate between bacteria and host membranes. Alternatively, AMPs can either specifically target the bacterial cell wall or the intra-cellular components by a non-membrane-targeting method [33]. AMPs' important role as a natural treatment against *S. aureus* is supported by findings that some commensal skin bacteria strains, including CoNS that produce AMPs against *S. aureus*, are deficient in the skin of AD patients. Replacing the deficient AMPs from commensal bacteria may help in treating the disease [35].

Human β-defensins (hBDs), another type of AMPs localized mainly in the skin and other epithelial surfaces, are often under-expressed in the skin of AD patients upon inflammation, leading to a greater likelihood of skin infection, such as by *S. aureus* [36]. Although conflicting study results about the dysregulation of hBD peptide levels exist, the decrease in mRNA level is identified in AD, indicating the active synthesis of hBDs is reduced [37, 38]. Furthermore, even if the levels of hBD-3 present in keratinocytes are similar in both normal and AD skin, a functional deficiency of keratinocyte-produced hBDs (specifically, hBD-3) derived from AD patients to control *S. aureus*, occurs [39].

Similarly, there is a deficiency of the AMP LL-37 in AD skin. The cathelicidin LL-37 contains 37 amino acids and, unlike hBDs, is expressed in epithelial surfaces, such as epidermal keratinocytes and intestinal cells, as well as non-epithelial areas such as in immune cells (e.g., T cells) and in body fluids [19]. Not only may LL-37 by itself be able to defend against pathogens such as *S. aureus*, but LL-37 was additionally found to produce an enhanced antimicrobial response when combined with prokaryotic AMPs from the commensal bacteria *S. hominis*, indicating a synergy between human and bacteria AMPs [35]. Conflicting study results about LL-37 expression in AD patients exist, and additional research is needed for LL-37 replacement to be considered as a future treatment option for AD [40, 41].

AMP deficiency is also connected to the anti-viral immune response. In one study of AD, ten patients with eczema herpeticum (EH), a serious and widespread skin infection that affects certain patients with AD upon infection with herpes simplex virus, and ten AD patients with no history of EH, those with EH history were found to have a significantly decreased level of LL-37 expression compared to non-EH AD patients, indicating a decreased immune defense against herpes virus infection for LL-37-deficient AD patients [42]. A similar study evaluated the experimentally induced expressions of hBD-2, hBD3, and LL-37 in nine AD patients with EH history. This study found relatively less induction in mRNAs corresponding to the three AMPs in lesional skin of EH patients versus nonlesional skin and lower induction compared to the skin of patients with psoriasis or AD without EH history [43].

Currently available AD treatment options include emollients; topical antibiotics; systemic immunosuppressants; topical corticosteroids; UV radiation; topical calcineurin inhibitors; and, most recently, anti-inflammatory biologics such as dupilumab [6, 7]. Recently, various studies on AD have provided evidence of therapeutic options aiming to correct disease-related barrier defects. Restoration of defective or deficient macromolecules or commensal bacteria in AD patients' skin may be a better treatment option. First, these replacement therapies may provide a physical and immune barrier as well as restoring the skin microenvironment and specifically targeting a cause of AD, rather than simply targeting symptoms such as inflammation. Moreover, restoring what is defective decreases the chance of adverse effects, such as epidermal thinning and atrophy with topical steroids or allergic reactions from synthetic products [44]. Furthermore, restoration therapy would, over time, be more eco-friendly, as fewer synthetic medications would be produced, used, and disposed of into the environment.

THE TECHNOLOGY OF SKIN BARRIER REGENERATION

Physical Barrier Restoration

Multiple studies have shown the viability of the restoration therapies discussed earlier. In terms of physical barrier repair, experts in the field have suggested that restoration of filaggrin or lipids such as ceramide may be used as a treatment for AD [8, 12, 45]. An animal model study supports the possibility of filaggrin replacement, as transepidermal delivery of cell-penetrating peptide (CPP)-linked recombinant filaggrin has resulted in the internalization of filaggrin and barrier function restoration [46]. Restoration of deficient lipids in the skin barrier has been studied in multiple randomized controlled trials, including some that specifically documented the positive effects of the application of a ceramide-containing emollient on risk of AD development [47, 48]. As for TJ, its critical role in the pathogenesis of AD still remains to be established.

Commensal Bacteria Restoration

Commensal bacteria restoration in both human patients and animal models has been shown to help in treating or even curing various diseases related to dysbiosis [22]. The same has been seen in patients with AD. Topically transplanting human commensal bacteria (such as *Roseomonas mucosa*) from healthy individuals to AD patients has been shown to decrease AD disease severity and decrease the need for topical steroids, with reduction of *S. aureus* [49]. Application of topical probiotics to AD skin has also been shown to improve skin barrier function and thus has a potential use as a treatment for AD patients, and the oral administration of probiotics has also resulted in a reduction of AD lesions in an animal model [50, 51].

AMP Restoration

Various methods have been studied or proposed as potential pathways for AMP restoration. Since CoNS, such as *S. epidermis* and *S. hominis*, produce AMPs with antimicrobial action against *S. aureus* and have shown to decrease *S. aureus* colonization in both a mouse model and human AD patients, topical transplantation of certain CoNS strains may help restore the skin microbiome and directly counter *S. aureus* with AMPs [35]. Additionally, the fact that conventional antimicrobials link to increase resistance to *S. aureus* in children with AD supports restoration treatments such as AMPs, which are less likely to lead to antibacterial resistance, for AD patients, especially as some *S. aureus* strains are resistant to almost all known conventional antibiotics [31, 32, 34, 50, 52].

UNFINISHED BUSINESS: CHALLENGES OF RESTORATION THERAPY

Medical researchers face many challenges before any of the potential treatments discussed in this chapter become commercially available. In general, any topically applied medications must be stable over time, bioavailable, effective, and safe.

Regulation Challenges

As medications that need to penetrate the stratum corneum (such as FLG and AMPs) are considered transdermal drug delivery systems, they would need to go through long-term preclinical toxicology studies, drug development, and multiple clinical trials, such as phase I for safety, phase II for dose finding and efficacy determination, and phase III for large-scale efficacy studies, before being submitted to the FDA for approval. Moreover, only a large market potential would provide sufficient incentive for pharmaceutical companies to undertake these costly drug development and clinical studies steps.

Formulation Challenges

One major challenge is that the effectiveness of topical application of biomacromolecules on the skin may be limited by the skin's poor permeability (with low permeability to nearly all molecules greater than 500 Da). Thus, traditional treatments often are unable to penetrate the stratum corneum [53]. One possible solution is the use of a CPP, which may serve as a skin penetration enhancer and facilitate application of macromolecules on the skin [54].

Although use of CPPs for transdermal delivery is relatively new, studies such as the CPP IMT-P8 in mouse skin and human tumor cells as well as successful internalization of a functional filaggrin monomer linked to a CPP to mouse and human epidermal tissue show that CPP may be a useful formulation option [46, 53].

Allergy and Autoimmunity Challenges

Although replacing what is deficient and already present in normal skin would decrease the chances of an allergic reaction, it is still possible for an allergic reaction to occur. Restoring a missing skin component due to genetic mutation could also induce an autoimmune reaction. Methods that can limit these possibilities should be investigated.

Technical Challenges of Physical Barrier Repair

Though replacement of topically applied recombinant filaggrin has been studied in a cell culture and an *in vivo* mouse model, comprehensive study into filaggrin restoration as a treatment for human AD patients would be needed [46]. Since this animal model has proven the ability of FLG restoration to be safely and functionally incorporated into the stratum corneum using a CPP, a similar method could also be applied to human skin lacking filaggrin, though more studies regarding frequency and quantity of application, which may depend on the degree of deficiency in an individual AD patient, are needed [46].

Furthermore, the cost of producing FLG is currently high; for example, 1 mg of *E. coli*-produced recombinant human filaggrin is priced at USD 1,215 by one biotechnology supplier as of July 2020 (Mybiosource. com, San Diego, CA). Additionally, although lipids such as ceramide are often present in many commercially available emollients, many of which are marketed for AD or eczema, more research is needed to determine the frequency of application, the rate of ceramide degradation, and the appropriate amount to achieve an optimal therapeutic result. Also noted, defects in the FLG gene are only present in roughly 20% to 50% of patients with AD, so barrier repair through restoration of FLG is not suitable for every AD patient [5, 12, 55, 56].

Technical Challenges of Reversal of Skin Dysbiosis

Generally, only limited evidence is available as to whether probiotics are successfully used for AD [7]. Additional research is needed to evaluate this treatment's effectiveness, frequency, and duration of application for AD patients.

Various bacteria species or strains have been evaluated or proposed for possible treatment, such as *R. mucosa*, *Lactobacillus rhamnosus* (especially *L. rhamnosus GG*), *Lactobacillus salivarius*, *Lactobacillus paracasei*, *Bifidobacterium breve*, *Bifidobacterium longum*, *Staphylococcus hominis*, and *Staphylococcus epidermis* [7, 35, 49]. However, additional research is needed to examine which species or strains would work best as a potential treatment for AD and the method by which they would best be applied to the skin, which may vary based on an individual's AD severity or skin microbiome composition. Additionally, the production of biofilms on AD skin by the pathogen *S. aureus* may pose a challenge, as they may prevent commensal bacteria from successfully colonizing the skin [21].

Technical Challenges of AMP Restoration Therapy

Despite the many advantages, challenges involving delivery, bioavailability, and production cost will need to be solved to ensure the efficacy and practicality of AMP restoration therapy [31, 57]. The delivery and bioavailability of AMPs may be improved through the use of different delivery systems, such as nanotube or nanoparticle-based technology, if applicable to skin, although some may still need to be tested more extensively for efficacy and potential side effects [57]. Though numerous peptide-based drugs have been approved and are currently available on the market, no synthetic AMPs have been approved yet, showing a need for more research into the use of AMPs as a treatment for AD and the corresponding delivery systems [58]. Another major challenge is that of a high production cost at an industrial scale, compared to conventional antibiotics. This calls for new methods and advances to lower the cost of AMPs. The use of nanotechnology or other delivery systems may also add cost due to the need for more research to increase stability, to reduce toxicity, and to limit side effects [31, 58].

Even as AMPs do have an advantage over conventional antibiotics in that they do not as readily result in antibiotic resistance, there have been cases recorded in which pathogenic bacteria do develop resistance to AMPs [34]. *S. aureus* has been specifically known to develop resistance to various AMPs by cleaving the AMP using protease, inactivating the AMP through binding, or using efflux pumps [32]. Additional research is needed to find effective ways, if any, to counter AMP resistance in bacteria if AMPs are to be used as treatments for AD in the future. Methods to counter the challenges of using AMPs are being considered. For example, recombinant techniques to produce AMPs may use eukaryotic organisms instead of single-cellular organisms, as they are less impacted by the AMPs' toxic effects, or use a carrier protein such as calmodulin to counter both AMP degradation and toxicity [31].

SUMMARY

The novel approaches to regenerate a healthy skin barrier in defected AD skin by topically applied regimens, particularly in eco-friendly ways, are supported by preliminary data. More work is needed before they can become approved therapies. See further Figure 7.1.

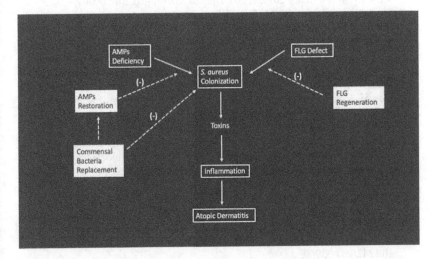

FIGURE 7.1 Regeneration of natural skin barrier for atopic dermatitis: a proposed strategy. (Solid arrows indicate disease-triggering influences. Dotted arrows depict countering effects of the regenerative therapies.)

REFERENCES

1. Sonkoly E, Muller A, Lauerma AI, et al. IL-31: A new link between T cells and pruritus in atopic skin inflammation. *J Allergy Clin Immunol* 2006; 117: 411–417. Doi: 10.1016/j.jaci.2005.10.033.

2. Fuxench ZCC, Block JK, Boguniewicz, M, et al. Atopic dermatitis in America study: A cross-sectional study examining the prevalence and disease burden of atopic dermatitis in the US adult population. *J Invest Dermatol* 2019; 139(3): 583–590. Doi: 10.1016/j.jid.2018.08.028.

3. Drucker AM, Wang AR, Li WQ, et al. The burden of atopic dermatitis: Summary of a report for the national eczema association. *J Invest Dermatol* 2017; 137(1): 26–30. Doi: 10.1016/j.jid.2016.07.012.

4. Schneider L, Hanifin J, Boguniewicz M, et al. Study of the atopic march: Development of atopic comorbidities. *Pediatr Dermatol* 2016; 33(4): 388–398. Doi: 10.1111/pde.12867.

5. Rerknimitr P, Otsuka A, Nakashima C, et al. The etiopathogenesis of atopic dermatitis: Barrier disruption, immunological derangement, and pruritis. *Inflammation and Regeneration* 2017; 37: 14. Doi: 10.1186/s41232-017-0044-7.

6. Kim J, Kim BE and Leung DYM. Pathophysiology of atopic dermatitis: Clinical implications. *Allergy Asthma Proc* 2019; 40: 84–92. Doi: 10.2500/aap.2019.40.4202.

7. Rather IA, Bajpai VK, Kumar S, et al. Probiotics and atopic dermatitis: An overview. *Front Microbiol* 2016; 7: 507. Doi: 10.3389/fmicb.2016.00507.

8. Kim BE and Leung DYM. Significance of skin barrier dysfunction in atopic dermatitis. *Allergy Asthma Immunol Res* 2018; 10(3): 207–215. Doi: 10.4168/aair.2018.10.3.207.

9. Yang G, Seok JK, Kang HC, et al. Skin barrier abnormalities and immune dysfunction in atopic dermatitis. *J Mol Sci* 2020; 21: 2867. Doi: 10.3390/ijms21082867.

10. Han H, Roan F, and Ziegler SF. The atopic march: Current insights into skin barrier dysfunction and epithelial cell-derived cytokines. *Immunol Rev* 2017; 278(1): 116–130. Doi: 10.1111/imr.12546.

11. Bao L, Mohan GC, Alexander JB, et al. A molecular mechanism for IL-4 suppression of loricrin transcription in epidermal keratinocytes: Implication for atopic dermatitis pathogenesis. *Innate Immun* 2017; 23(8): 641–647. Doi: 10.1177/1753425917732823.

12. Agrawal R and Woodfolk JA. Skin barrier defects in atopic dermatitis. *Curr Allergy Asthma Rep* 2014; 14(5): 433. Doi: 10.1007/s11882-014-0433-9.

13. Sandilands A, Sutherland C, Irvine AD, et al. Filaggrin in the frontline: Role in skin barrier function and disease. *J Cell Sci* 2009; 122(9): 1285–1294. Doi: 10.1242/jcs.033969.

14. Bantz SK, Zhu Z, and Zheng T. The atopic march: Progression from atopic dermatitis to allergic rhinitis and asthma. *J Clin Cell Immunol* 2014; 5(2): 202. Doi: 10.4172/2155-9899.1000202.

15. Ziyab AH, Karmaus W, Zhang H, et al. Association of filaggrin variants with asthma and rhinitis: Is eczema or allergic sensitization status an effect modifier? *Int Arch Allergy Immunol* 2014; 164(4): 308–318. Doi: 10.1159/000365990.

16. Li S, Villarreal M, Stewart S, et al. Altered composition of epidermal lipids correlates with *Staphylococcus aureus* colonization status in atopic dermatitis. *Br J Dermatol* 2017; 177(4): e125–e127. Doi: 10.1111/bjd.15409.

17. De Benedetto A, Rafaels NM, McGirt LY, et al. Tight junction defects in atopic dermatitis. *J Allergy Clin Immunol* 2010; 127(3): 773–786.e7. Doi: 10.1016/j.jaci.2010.10.018.

18. Furuse M, Hata M, Furuse K, et al. Claudin-based tight junctions are crucial for the mammalian epidermal barrier: A lesson from claudin-1-deficient mice. *J Cell Biol* 2002; 156(6): 1099–1111. Doi: 10.1083/jcb.200110122.

19. Hata TR and Gallo RL. Antimicrobial peptides, skin infections and atopic dermatitis. *Semin Cutan Med Surg* 2008; 27(2): 144–150. Doi: 10.1016/j.sder.2008.04.002.

20. Paller AS, Kong HH, Seed P, et al. The microbiome in patients with atopic dermatitis. *J Allergy Clin Immunol* 2019; 143(1): 26–35. Doi: 10.1016/j.jaci.2018.11.015.

21. Di Domenico EG, Cavallo I, Capitano B, et al. *Staphylococcus aureus* and the cutaneous microbiota biofilms in the pathogenesis of atopic dermatitis. *Microorganisms* 2019; 7(9): 301. Doi: 10.3390/microorganisms7090301.

22. Petersen C and Round RL. Defining dysbiosis and its influence on host immunity and disease. *Cellular Microbiol* 2014; 16(7): 1024–1033. Doi: 10.1111/cmi.12308.

23. Nakatsuji T and Gallo RL. The role of the skin microbiome in atopic dermatitis. *Ann Allergy Asthma Immunol* 2019; 263–269. https://doi.org/10.1016/j.anai.2018.12.003.

24. Balato A, Cacciapuoti S, Di Caprio R, et al. Human microbiome: Composition and role in inflammatory skin diseases. *Archivum Immunologiae et Therapiae Experimentalis* 2019; 67: 1–18. https://doi.org/10.1007/s00005-018-0528-4.

25. Honda K and Littman DR. The microbiota in adaptive immune homeostasis and disease. *Nature* 2016; 535(7610): 75–84. Doi: 10.1038/nature18848.

26. Kennedy EA, Connoly J, Hourihane JOB, et al. Skin microbiome before development of atopic dermatitis: Early colonization with commensal staphylococci at 2 months is associated with a lower risk of atopic dermatitis at 1 year. *J Allergy Clin Immunol* 2017; 139(1): 166–172. Doi: 10.1016/j.jaci.2016.07.029.

27. Meylan P, Lang C, Mermoud S, et al. Skin colonization by *Staphylococcus aureus* precedes the clinical diagnosis of atopic dermatitis in infancy. *Journal of Investigative Dermatology* 2017; 137: 2497–2504. Doi: 10.1016/j.jid.2017.07.834.

28. Park KD, Pak SC, and Park KK. The pathogenic effect of natural and bacterial toxins on atopic dermatitis. *Toxins (Basel)* 2017; 9(1): 3. Doi: 10.3390/toxins9010003.

29. Kong HH, Oh J, Deming C, et al. Temporal shifts in the skin microbiome associated with disease flares and treatment in children with atopic dermatitis. *Genome Res* 2012; 22(5): 850–859. Doi: 10.1101/gr.131029.111.

30. Byrd AL, Deming C, Cassidy SKB, et al. *Staphyloccocus aureus* and *Staphyloccocus epidermis* strain diversity underlying pediatric atopic dermatitis. *Sci Transl Med* 2017; 9(937): eaal4651. Doi: 10.1126/scitranslmed.aal4651.

31. Boto A, Pérez de la Lastra JM and González CC. The road from host-defense peptides to a new generation of antimicrobial drugs. *Molecules* 2018; 23(2): 311. Doi: 10.3390/molecules23020311.

32. Moravej H, Moravej Z, Yazdanparast M, et al. Antimicrobial peptides: Features, action, and their resistance mechanisms in bacteria. *Microb Drug Resist* 2018; 24(6): 747–767. https://doi.org/10.1089/mdr.2017.0392.

33. Kumar P, Kizhakkedathu JN, and Straus SK. Antimicrobial peptides: Diversity, mechanism of action and strategies to improve the activity and biocompatibility in vivo. *Biomolecules* 2018; 8(4). Doi: 10.3390/biom8010004.

34. Pfalzgraff A, Brandenburg K, and Günther W. Antimicrobial peptides and their therapeutic potential for bacterial skin infections and wounds. *Front Pharmacol* 2018. Doi: 10.3389/fphar.2018.00281.

35. Nakatsuji T, Chen TH, Narala S, et al. Antimicrobials from human skin commensal bacteria protect against *Staphylococcus aureus* and are deficient in atopic dermatitis. *Sci Transl Med* 2017; 9(378). Doi: 10.1126/scitranslmed. aah4680.

36. Chieosilapatham P, Ogawa H, and Niyonsaba F. Current insights into the role of human β-defensins in atopic dermatitis. *Clinical and Experimental Immunology* 2017. Doi: 10.1111/cei.13013.

37. Clausen ML, Jungersted JM, Andersen PS, et al. Human β-defensin-2 as a marker for disease severity and skin barrier properties in atopic dermatitis. *Br J Dermatol* 2013; 169(3): 587–598. Doi: 10.1111/bjd.12419.

38. Noh YH, Lee J, Seo SJ, et al. Promoter DNA methylation contributes to human β-defensin-1 deficiency in atopic dermatitis. *Anim Cells Syst (Seoul)* 2018; 22(3): 172–177. Doi: 10.1080/19768354.2018.1458652.

39. Kisich KO, Carspecken CW, Fiéve S, et al. Defective killing of staphylococcus aureus in atopic dermatitis is associated with reduced mobilization of human beta-defensin-3. *J Allergy Clin Immunol* 2008; 122(1): 62–68. Doi: 10.1016/j. jacl.1008.04.022.

40. Kanda N, Hau CS, Tada Y, et al. Decreased serum LL-37 and vitamin D3 levels in atopic dermatitis: Relationship between IL-31 and oncostatin M. *Allergy* 2012; 67(6): 804–812. Doi: 10.1111/j.1398-9995.2012.02824.x.

41. Ballardini N, Johansson C, Lilja G, et al. Enhanced expression of the antimicrobial peptide LL-37 in lesional skin of adults with atopic eczema. *Br J Dermatol* 2009; 161(1): 40–47. Doi: 10.1111/j.1365-2133.2009.09095.x.

42. Howell MD, Wollenberg A, Gallo RL, et al. Cathelicidin deficiency predisposes to eczema herpeticum. *J Allergy Clin Immunol* 2006; 117(4): 836–841. Doi: 10.1016/j.jaci.2005.12.1345.

43. Hata TR, Kotol P, Boguniewicz M, et al. History of eczema herpeticum is associated with the ability to induce human β-defensin (HBD)-2, HBD-3 and cathelicidin in the skin of patients with atopic dermatitis. *Br J Dermatol* 2010; 163(3): 659–661. Doi: 10.1111/j.1365-2133.2010.09892.x.

44. Bower AJ, Arp Z, Zhao Y, et al. Longitudinal *in vivo* tracking of adverse effects following topical steroid treatment. *Exp Dermatol* 2016; 25(5): 362–367. Doi: 10.1111/exd.12932.

45. Brown SJ and McLean WHI. One remarkable molecule: Filaggrin. *J Invest Dermatol* 2012; 132(3 Pt 2): 751–762. Doi: 10.1038/jid.2011.393.

46. Stout TE, McFarland T, Mitchell JC, et al. Recombinant filaggrin is internalized and processed to correct filaggrin deficiency. *J Invest Dermatol* 2014; 134: 423–429. Doi: 10.1038/jid.2013.284.
47. Lowe A, Su J, Tang M, et al. PEBBLES study protocol: A randomised controlled trial to prevent atopic dermatitis, food allergy, and sensitisation in infants with a family history of allergic disease using a skin barrier improvement strategy. *BMJ Open* 2019; 9(3): e024594. Doi: 10.1136/bmjopen-2018-024594.
48. McClanahan D, Wong A, Kezic S, et al. A randomized control trial of an emollient with ceramide and filaggrin-associated amino acids for the primary prevention of atopic dermatitis in high-risk infants. *J Eur Acad Dermatol Venereol* 2019; Doi: 10.1111/jdv.15786.
49. Myles IA, Earland NJ, Andersen ED, et al. First-in-human microbiome transplantation with *Roseomonas mucosa* for atopic dermatitis. *JCI Insight* 2018. https://doi.org/10.1172/jci.insight.120608.
50. Marcinkowska M, Zagórska A, Fajkis N, et al. A review of probiotic supplementation and feasibility of topical application for the treatment of pediatric atopic dermatitis. *Curr Pharm Biotechnol* 2018; 19(10): 827–838. Doi: 10.2174/138920 1019666181008113149.
51. Kim WK, Jang YJ, Han DH, et al. *Lactobacillus paracasei* KBL382 administration attenuates atopic dermatitis by modulating immune response and gut microbiota. *Gut Microbiota* 2020. https://doi.org/10.1080/19490976.202 0.1819156.
52. Harkins CP, McAleer MA, Bennett D, et al. The widespread use of topical antimicrobials enriches resistance in *Staphylococcus aureus* isolated from patients with atopic dermatitis. *Br J Dermatol* 2018; 179: 807–808. Doi: 10.1111/ bjd.16722.
53. Gautam A, Nanda JS, Samuel JS, et al. Topical delivery of protein and peptide using novel cell penetrating peptide IMT-P8. *Sci Rep* 2016; 6: 26278. Doi: 10.1038/srep26278.
54. Tan J, Cheong H, Park, YS, et al. Cell-penetrating peptide-mediated topical delivery of biomacromolecular drugs. *Curr Pharm Biotechnoll* 2015; 15(3): 231–239. Doi: 10.2174/1389201015666140614094320.
55. Palmer CNA, Irvine AD, Terron-Kwiatkowski A, et al. Common loss-of-function variants of the epidermal barrier protein filaggrin are a major predisposing factor for atopic dermatitis. *Nature Genetics* 2006; 38: 441–446.
56. On HR, Lee SE, Kim SE, et al. Filaggrin mutation in Korean patients with atopic dermatitis. *Yonsei Med J* 2017; 58(2): 395–400. Doi: 10.3349/ymj.2017.58.2.395.
57. Piotrowska U, Sobczak M, and Oledzka E. Current state of a dual behaviour of antimicrobial peptides: Therapeutic agents and promising delivery vectors. *Chemical Biology & Drug Design* 2017. https://doi.org/10.1111/cbdd.13031.
58. Biswaro LS, da Costa Sousa MG, Rezende TMB, et al. Antimicrobial peptides and nanotechnology, recent advances and challenges. *Front Microbiol* 2018; 9: 855. Doi: 10.3389/fmicb.2018.00855.

PART III

Speed Cutaneous Medicine

Mohs Micrographic Surgery *sine* Microscopy

8

The Winning Speed of Mass Spectrometry

Lawrence S. Chan

Contents

DOI: 10.1201/9781003121275-11

INTRODUCTION

Mohs micrographic surgery, commonly referred as Mohs surgery, was initially developed by Dr. Fredric Mohs, an otolaryngologist at the University of Wisconsin. The original procedure, initially termed chemosurgery, was performed with a zinc chloride–based paste to destroy cancerous tissue layer by layer under microscopic control [1]. Subsequently, Mohs surgery was modified to the present and widely accepted form, in part to eliminate the pain associated with zinc chloride and in part to improve efficiency [2]. The refined procedure currently performed by Mohs surgeons consists four major steps: 1) the removal of a layer of clinically visible skin cancer (with small surrounding healthy tissue) from the patient; 2) the cryo-sectioning and staining of the removed skin layer marked with orientation; 3) the microscopic examination of the stained cryo-sections for the presence of cancer at its margins, repeating the first three steps if a positive margin is detected; and 4) the repair of the surgical wound by a skin surgical technique called flap [3]. The two goals of Mohs surgery are to remove cancer with the greatest certainty and to preserve healthy tissue to the maximum extent. For this reason, the Mohs surgery technique is utilized the most for surgery performed on skin cancer occurring in head and neck locations, for which preserving healthy tissue and clearing cancer are both essential. These two goals are especially critical when skin cancer surfaces near vital organs, such as eye, nose, mouth, and ear, since tissue preservation is essential for the functional integrity of these organs, and tumor clearance is important to eliminate cancer recurrence and spread to involve these organs. Not surprisingly, Mohs surgery has achieved a high cure rate for skin cancers while helping physicians achieve maximum preservation of healthy tissue. A professional guideline provides a road map for the appropriate use of the Mohs technique to physicians in approaching patients they encounter [4]. Recently, an emerging biomedical analytical technique with mass spectrometry (MS) has been developed to perform intraoperative cancer margin determination. It has the potential to revolutionize the Mohs micrographic surgery by eliminating the need for microscopic examination in the future; hence, this chapter discusses the proposed "Mohs micrographic surgery *sine* microscopy" [5–7].

ANALYSIS OF THE NEED

Having defined the technical steps of currently performed Mohs micrographic surgery, we now look into the need for improving the speed of the procedure. A 2006 study estimated that there were 3.5 million new cases of non-melanoma skin cancers occurring in the US, and this number is likely to be an annual-occurrence figure [8]. The same research team reported that the overall procedures performed for non-melanoma skin cancers increased by 14% from 2006 to 2012 and that the estimated incidence was 4 million cases in 2012 [9]. The majority of non-melanoma skin cancers are basal cell carcinomas and squamous cell carcinomas. Approximately, one out of four skin cancers are treated by Mohs surgery [4]. The current practice of Mohs micrographic surgery, though it serves the medical community well by providing a substantial possibility of cure for the detected cancer while maximally preserving healthy skin in the critical facial locations, is a very labor-intense procedure. It requires a Mohs surgeon to remove a layer of cancer-present skin, a pathology tech to perform cryo-sectioning and staining, and a Mohs surgeon to examine the clearance of the cancer at the tissue margins under a microscope. Moreover, it is a time-consuming process. The patient must sit and wait for the microscopic determination whether the excised tissue is indeed cancer-free. If the initial excision layer did not clear the skin cancer (i.e., the layer examined under microscope contains positive cancer at one of its margins), the process repeats all over again: another layer of skin removed, another round of frozen section cut and stained, and then another round of stained sections examined microscopically. The procedure will continue as necessary until all margins are clear. At this point, the Mohs surgeon can then proceed to close the wound using a technique termed flap, which essentially is to move a piece of connected healthy skin adjacent to the wound to cover the surgical defect. A substantial amount of time in the entire Mohs procedure is spent in the determination of the cancer margin: cutting frozen sections, staining, and microscopic examination. Therefore, an innovative approach to shorten the time spent on the cancer margin determination portion would significantly reduce the time needed for the procedure. Enter the speed of MS!

PRINCIPLE OF MS

Before discussing the Mohs procedure with MS, it is useful to get some basic understanding of the MS technology itself [10, 11]. The operational principles of MS follow three key steps: ionization, analysis (acceleration and deflection), and detection.

Ionization

In order for a molecule to be properly analyzed by MS, the molecule must be ionized. The most common type of ionization is an electro form. Then the sample, which is vaporized, is sent through a chamber, where it will be bombarded by electrons from a heated filament. The high energy of the electrons in the chamber knocks out the electrons of the sample, forming ions of the sample.

Analysis: Acceleration and Deflection

After the first step of ionization, the ionized molecule is then sorted according to its mass-to-charge ratio in two stages: acceleration and deflection. In the acceleration stage, the ionized molecule is placed between a set of charged parallel plates and will be repelled by one plate and attracted to the other.

In the deflection stage, the ions are passed through the magnetic field and deflected to the detector. The amount of deflection is dependent on the mass and charge of the molecule. The lighter ions and ions with positive charge of 1 are deflected the most, whereas the heavier ions or ions with a positive charge of 2 or larger are deflected the least.

Detection

Finally, the molecule will be detected by MS for its mass-to-charge ratio (symbol m/z) and relative abundance. When the ion reaches the detector, it will be neutralized by electrons and its signal sent to be amplified and then to be recognized by a computer that converts the signal to mass/charge ratio, and a spectrum is generated for visualization. The key usefulness of MS rests on the principle that the test molecule's m/z characterized by MS is a unique fingerprint of that particular molecule.

It is well known that cancer cells frequently contain unique gene products and the corresponding metabolites. Since cancer-specific metabolites commonly exhibit distinct *m/z* compared to healthy tissue metabolites, either qualitatively or quantitatively, MS could be valuable for intraoperative cancer determination.

THE TECHNOLOGY FOR INTRAOPERATIVE MARGIN DETECTION

Several recent publications have documented the usefulness of MS as an intraoperative margin detection tool, replacing the microscopic method [12]. The following section discusses two clinical examples.

Intraoperative Margin Detection for Brain Tumors

In an effort to develop a rapid method of intraoperative margin detection, researchers at Harvard Medical School and its affiliated medical centers looked into the possibility of using desorption electrospray ionization (DESI) MS for the purpose of mapping brain tumor margins during surgery. The impetus for such investigative efforts included the following [12]:

- The currently employed microscopic method, which was developed more than 150 years ago, is time consuming, taking 30 minutes for the preparation of slides, staining, and examination.
- The currently employed H & E staining of frozen tissue sections frequently produces processing artifacts, thus interfering with accurate tumor determination under microscopy.
- Certain brain tumors, such as infiltrative gliomas, are difficult to visualize microscopically, contributing to the resulting suboptimal surgical excision and reduced patient survival.
- Certain brain tumors, such as gliomas, have been shown to harbor mutations in gene encoding isocitrate dehydrogenases 1 and 2, the enzymes capable of converting isocitrate to 2-hydroxyglutarate (2-HG).
- The tumor-specific metabolite 2-HG is highly concentrated in tumor tissues, compared to its minimal presence in normal tissues, giving

a distinct quantitative marker critically useful in MS-directed detection of brain tumors.

- The MS-directed detection method operates at room (ambient) temperature, thus providing another convenience factor.
- The MS-directed method does not destroy the tissue sample if a histologically compatible solvent is used, providing the opportunity to correlate the MS findings with those of histology.

The Harvard researchers studies subsequently determined that [12]:

- A correlation is established between the intensity of the 2-HG signal and the concentration of tumor cells in the specimens.
- DESI MS detects 2-HG signals with greater sensitivity than immunohistochemistry, as some isocitrate dehydrogenases mutations occur in uncommon protein locations, resulting in conformational changes that reduce the ability of binding by the monoclonal antibodies supplied in the immunohistochemistry kits.
- The DESI MS two-dimensional image of 2-HG spatial molecular data can be overlaid onto the optical image of H & E-stained tissue, forming a discriminatory capacity to define the tumor margin.
- DESI MS molecular data can be three-dimensionally mapped onto an MRI-constructed tumor location, thus providing the possibility of avoiding interrupting intraoperative MRI during surgery.
- In a real-life patient brain operation, a swab of excisional tissue sample enables the DESI MS to detect, within minutes, the tumor-specific metabolite 2-HG (with a *m/z* peak of 147.0). This finding is later confirmed by the gene mutations of isocitrate dehydrogenases by the immunohistochemistry method.

A Handheld MS System for Intraoperative Cancer Detection

Researchers from the University of Texas at Austin and colleagues at Baylor College of Medicine and MD Anderson Cancer Center examined a handheld MS system for its usefulness in intraoperative cancer margin detection, and they established the following [5]:

- A handheld device or probe, called a "MasSpec Pen," is optimized to contain three conduits: 1) an incoming port that delivers a single water droplet to the device's tip, 2) a central port that delivers inert gas, and 3) an outgoing port that delivers the water droplet–contained molecules extracted from the tissue to the MS system for analysis.

- When connected to a DESI MS system, the MasSpec Pen can provide a controlled and automated delivery of water droplets at its tip for efficient extraction of biomolecules on the tissue surface for MS analysis without tissue destruction. When the probe tip touches the sample tissue, a water droplet is delivered and remains on the tip for three seconds, time sufficient for molecule extraction. When the probe is removed from the sample tissue, the opening of conduit 3 allows the vacuum extraction of the molecule-containing droplet to the MS system for analysis. The inert gas provides a stabilizing force to prevent tubing collapse during vacuum extraction.

- The MasSpec Pen MS system can obtain rapid diagnostic information for cancer at the tissue margin. The entire process from touching the tissue with the MasSpec probe to the acquisition of MS data (*m/z* peak) is accomplished within ten seconds.

- Using *ex vivo* molecular analysis of 20 human cancer thin-tissue sections and 253 human patient samples of normal and cancerous tissues, the MS system collects a large database of biomarkers, enabling an artificial intelligence–directed statistical classifier built from the histologically validated molecular database to perform cancer prediction.

- The MS system achieves high sensitivity (96.4%), specificity (96.2%), and overall accuracy (96.3%).

- Performing on an *in vivo* breast cancer–bearing mouse model, the MS system with MasSpec Pen demonstrates its suitability in cancer margin detection, without causing physical harm or stress to the tested animals.

Mohs Micrographic Surgery *sine* Microscopy: A Proposal

Having illustrated the usefulness of MS for intraoperative cancer margin determination in brain cancer surgery and the high-performance capability of a handheld MS device (MasSpec Pen), the following delineate the proposed operative approach for the future "Mohs micrographic surgery *sine* microscopy" for skin cancers [7].

Step 1. Removal by the Mohs surgeon of a layer of clinically visible skin cancer (along with a minimum 1 mm margin of healthy skin). This step is identical to the currently practiced procedure.

Step 2. The Mohs surgeon marks the orientation of the removed skin layer and the corresponding wound edge so as to identify the location in case additional removal is indicated. This step is identical to the currently practiced procedure.

Step 3. The Mohs surgeon or his/her assistant covers the patient's wound and lets the patient rest on the operating table. This step is different from the currently practiced procedure, since the patient will not need to rest in the waiting room as the cancer margin will be determined in just a few minutes.

Step 4. The Mohs surgeon examines the cancer margin of the removed tissue using a handheld MS device (MasSpec Pen). This step will replace the three currently practiced steps: 1) cutting and marking the sequential frozen tissue sections and placing them on glass slides, 2) staining the slide sections, and 3) examining all the stained sections for cancer presence at the margins under a microscope. The details as previously described [11] are depicted in Figure 8.1.

- The physician who performs the Mohs surgery will use the MasSpec Pen to gently touch the edges of the removed tissue in which the physician wants to rule out residual cancer.
- The water-soluble molecules, including tumor-specific metabolites, will be dissolved by water droplets suspended at the tip of the MasSpec Pen, mixed with inert gas, and pumped to a MS machine for analysis.
- The sample molecules in the droplet will be ionized and then analyzed in the mass spectrometer.

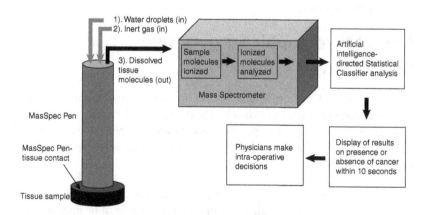

FIGURE 8.1   Intraoperative cancer detection by MasSpec Pen.

- The mass-to-charge ratios (*m/z*), unique fingerprints for each molecule, will be determined, and the information will be sent to an artificial intelligence–directed software called Statistical Classifier for determination. The AI-directed program, which has been previously trained and validated with 100 cancerous and healthy skin tissues, will send the signal back to the operating physician at nearly real-time speed (in few seconds), informing the physician if that tissue point of touch is positive or negative for cancer. The accuracy is generally greater than 95%. The physician continues to search all edges of the removed tissue and mark the areas of positive cancer presence for the next layer of removal. If cancer is found at one of the margins, steps 1 through 4 will be repeated until all margins are clear of the presence of cancer.

Step 5. Wound closure by Mohs surgeon with flaps when all edges of the removed layer are clear for cancer presence. This step is identical to the currently practiced procedure.

UNFINISHED BUSINESS

To develop a commercially viable and medically sound procedure, the following issues need to be resolved, and they are resolvable, provided that these conditions are met: sufficient patient base, sufficient financial investment, committed human effort, and clinic-size and affordable mass spectrometer.

Sufficient Patient Base

In order to identify the unique tumor metabolite in a particular skin cancer, there is a need for a sufficient number of patients. Similarly, in order to train and validate the artificial intelligence–directed Statistical Classifier program, a sufficient number of patients will also be needed. Such requirement can be achieved by the collective efforts of several collaborative medical centers.

Sufficient Financial Investment

Any new technical development requires substantial investment; the development of a new Mohs surgery procedure is no exception. These investments include both financial and human efforts. In the financial aspect, investment will be needed to support basic science and clinical research efforts. In the basic science equation, we need investment for identifying the molecular marker—likely a tumor-specific metabolite—that we can use to distinguish skin cancer from normal human skin tissue. Once the molecular marker is identified, the next step will be investment in the needed equipment: i.e., the mass spectrometer and the "MasSpec Pen" [5]. From the clinical research perspective, we need investment to support the validation of the "MasSpec Pen" in making correct skin cancer margin detection. These investment supports are needed for the physicians (Mohs surgeons), the artificial intelligence platform, and the pathologists who perform the histological validation.

Committed Human Effort

Financial investment alone without committed human effort would lead a development nowhere. Human effort will be needed to organize a collaborative team, including Mohs surgeons, pathologists, clinical research coordinators, AI computer scientists, mass spectrometry experts, and mass spectrometer company representatives. While mass spectrometer company representatives will provide the needed equipment (the mass spectrometer machine and MasSpec Pen), the other team members will be responsible for protocol development, patient recruitment, record keeping, result documenting, pathology validation, and AI data input and output adjustment.

Clinic-Size and Affordable Mass Spectrometer

In addition to the financial investment and human effort, we also need a reasonably small-size mass spectrometry machine that fits into an outpatient clinic setting. At the present time, a regular mass spectrometry machine is huge in size, thus making it a logistic impossibility to set up an outpatient surgical suite with this kind of machine. In addition, the purchase price of a regular-size mass spectrometer is close to US \$1 million, which is prohibitively expensive for a physician or even a physician group. Therefore, it may not be possible to democratize such microscope-less Mohs surgery until such time comes that a reasonably priced and size machine is available. A new generation of mass spectrometers manufactured by ThermoFisher Scientific Company (Model Orbitrap Exploris™ 240 Mass Spectrometer), with a footprint size about 21 inches by 30 inches and an approximate price tag of US \$250,000 will be a significant step forward to achieving a widely accepted application of Mohs micrographic surgery *sine* microscopy [13].

SUMMARY

Based on the up-to-date clinical evidence, MS can potentially be a game-changer for performing Mohs surgery by eliminating the need for the time-consuming steps of skin sectioning, staining, and microscopic examination. The future for wide adaptation of this technology will depend on additional human effort and financial investment.

REFERENCES

1. Mohs FE. *Chemosurgery: Microscopically Controlled Surgery for Skin Cancer.* Charles C. Thomas, Springfield, IL, 1978.
2. Tromovitch TA, Stegeman SJ. Microscopically controlled excision of skin tumors. *Arch Dermatol* 1974: 110L231–110L232.
3. Rohrer TE, Cook JL, Kaufman A. *Flaps and Grafts in Dermatologic Surgery.* 2nd Ed. Elsevier, Cambridge, MA, 2017.
4. Connolly SM, Baker DR, Coldiron BM, et al. AAD/ACMS/ASDSA/ASMS 2012 appropriate use criteria for Mohs micrographic surgery: A report of the American Academy of Dermatology, American College of Mohs Surgery, American Society for Dermatologic Surgery Association, and the American Society for Mohs Surgery. *J Am Acad Dermatol* 2012; 67(4): 531–550. Doi: 10.1016/j.jaad.2012.06.009.
5. Zhang J, Rector J, Lin JQ, et al. Nondestructive tissue analysis for ex vivo and in vivo cancer diagnosis using a handheld mass spectrometry system. *Sci Transl Med* 2017; 9(406): Doi: 10.1126/scitranslmed.aan3968.
6. Margulis K, Chiou AS, Aasi SZ, et al. Distinguishing malignant from benign microscopic skin lesions using desorption electrospray ionization mass spectrometry imaging. *Proc Natl Acad Sci USA* 2018; 115: 6347–6352.
7. Chan LS. Mohs micrographic surgery sine microscopy: Is mass spectrometry an upcoming intraoperative cancer margin assessment tool? *Ann Clin Oncol* 2019; 1(1): 1–3. http://dx.doi.org/10.31487/j.ACO.2018.01.06.
8. Rogers HW, Weinstock MA, Harris AR, et al. Incidence estimate of nonmelanoma skin cancer in the United States, 2006. *Arch Dermatol* 2010; 146: 283–287. Doi: 10.1001/archdermatol.2010.19.
9. Rogers HW, Weinstock MA, Feldman SR, et al. Incidence estimate of non-melanoma skin cancer (keratinocyte carcinomas) in the U.S. Population, 2012. *JAMA Dermatol* 2015; 151(10): 1081–1086. Doi: 10.1001/jamadermatol.2015.1187.
10. Urban PL. Quantitative mass spectrometry: An overview. *Philos Trans A Math Phys Eng Sci* 2016; 374(2079): 20150382. Doi: 10.1098/rsta.2015.0382.

11. Zhu R and Chan LS. Emerging biomedical analysis: Mass spectrometry. In: Chan LS and Tang WC. Eds. *Engineering-Medicine: Principles and Applications of Engineering in Medicine.* CRC Press, Boca Raton, FL, 2019; pp. 280–298.

12. Santagata S, Eberlin LS, Norton I, et al. Intraoperative mass spectrometry mapping of an onco-metabolite to guide brain tumor surgery. *Proc Natl Acad Sci USA* 2014; 111(30): 11121–11126.

13. [THERMOFISHER] Orbitrap exploris™ 240 mass spectrometer. ThermoFisher Scientific. [thermofisher.com/order/catalog/product/BRE725535#/BRE725535] Accessed June 19, 2020.

PART IV

Precision Cutaneous Medicine

Gene Editing Therapies for Genodermatoses

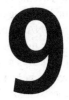

Adam Sheriff, Imogen Brooks, and Joanna Jacków

Contents

INTRODUCTION

Gene, or genome, editing is a therapy that directly corrects pathogenic mutations at the genomic level. By restoring normal gene and protein function in the skin, the disease is treated permanently. Gene editing typically creates a single- or double-strand break (DSB) in the DNA at a specific locus and uses the cell's endogenous repair mechanisms to introduce specific genetic

DOI: 10.1201/9781003121275-13

changes at this locus. When a DSB occurs, mammalian cells implement one of two mechanisms to repair their DNA: non-homologous end joining (NHEJ) or homology-directed repair (HDR). NHEJ-mediated repair joins blunt ends of DNA after DSBs and is more efficient, but it is error prone and tends to incur uncontrolled gene insertions or deletions (indels) at the site of the DSB [1, 2]. It is a robust method to disrupt genes and clinically useful in conditions where gene knockout is desirable, such as dominant negative mutations [1], or for exon-skipping [3]. HDR, on the other hand, engenders precise excision of the mutation using homologous recombination to incorporate endogenous or exogenous donor DNA for high-fidelity repair. HDR is favored for gene editing therapy that aims to reverse the disease genotype [4]. Alternatively, single-strand breaks and subsequent targeting of a base can lead to a change in the DNA sequence by cellular base-excision repair [5].

The skin is particularly suited for genome editing due to its accessibility for biopsy collection and treatment application [6]. Furthermore, skin can be easily visualized for the monitoring of positive or negative outcomes on gene-edited tissues (see Figure 9.1). Genodermatoses are rare inherited skin diseases that could be targeted for gene editing. Examples include epidermolysis bullosa (EB), which is a group of skin disorders that cause blistering, skin fragility, and occasionally systemic involvement [7]; some forms of ichthyosis; and Netherton syndrome. However, there are also more than 300 other genetic skin diseases, involving over 500 distinct genes [8, 9].

ANALYSIS OF THE NEED

Generally, treatments for genodermatoses are limited to symptom management with no curative potential or significant improvements in quality or length of life for patients. There is, therefore, an unmet need for new therapeutic options for patients with inherited skin diseases. Advances in molecular diagnostics have enabled identification of the mutations responsible for many genodermatoses, paving the way for gene editing therapies to permanently reverse them and cure the disease. Gene editing for genodermatoses can be compared to gene-addition therapy, which instead introduces an exogenous copy of a gene to recapitulate protein expression. Treating forms of EB has been clinically successful with gene addition [10–13]; however, challenges include inaccurate spatial-temporal gene expression, potential insertional mutagenesis or genotoxicity, aberrant splicing, and progressive extinction of the therapeutic transgene [1, 3, 6]. Protein, cell replacement, and RNA-based treatments are also being pursued but require ongoing treatment [14]. Gene editing provides a desirable alternative with long-term curative potential and physiological gene expression [15].

THE TECHNOLOGY

CRISPR-Cas Genome Editing

Historically, three major techniques—namely, meganucleases, zinc finger nucleases (ZFNs), and TALE nucleases (TALENs)—have been used for site-specific gene editing by introducing DSBs and using donor DNA to induce HDR [7]. However, in 2012, Jinek et al. uncovered a new strategy of genome editing that has several advantages over previous approaches [16]. Clustered regularly interspaced short palindromic repeat (CRISPR) sequences combined with a CRISPR-associated (Cas) nuclease protein enables targeting and manipulation of the genome with a high degree of specificity [8]. The CRISPR-Cas system evolved as a component of the immunity of bacteria and archaea [16], in which sequences from pathogens are transcribed into "CRISPR RNAs" (crRNAs) which then direct Cas endonucleases to institute a DSB at a specific DNA site on the invader, thus neutralizing it. Synthetic crRNAs called (single) guide RNAs ((s)gRNAs) can be developed to target Cas endonucleases to 20 nucleotide regions to create site-specific DNA cleavage on the genome. Synthesizing gRNAs for precision genome targeting is simpler, more affordable, and has greater scalability than reengineering protein recognition sites for ZFNs and TALENs [1, 6, 17]. "Multiplexing" is also feasible; multiple gRNAs are encoded to simultaneously edit several sites of the genome, supporting the wider applicability of the CRISPR-Cas9 system compared to previous technologies [17]. The type II CRISPR-Cas system, involving the Cas9 nuclease, is the best characterized and has been extensively studied since its first successful demonstration in mammalian cells [2, 17, 18].

The CRISPR-Cas9 system has been employed in several studies to target disease-causing mutations in different genodermatoses. EB is a prominent target for CRISPR-Cas9 editing due to its monogenic nature and well-described mechanism of disease. Classically, EB can be divided into three subtypes: EB simplex (EBS), junctional EB (JEB), and dystrophic EB (DEB), depending on the level of the skin at which blisters form. DEB is caused by mutations in the *COL7A1* gene, which leads to blisters in the superficial dermis due to deficiency of anchoring fibril (AF) function [7]. DEB can be inherited in either an autosomal dominant (DDEB) or recessive (RDEB) fashion. One study has shown the feasibility of NHEJ-dependent exon skipping to mitigate a recurrent RDEB frameshift mutation in *COL7A1* exon 80 [3]. NHEJ removed the mutation-bearing Exon 80 at 66.5% efficiency and subsequent skin grafting of edited keratinocytes onto mice demonstrated long-term restoration of phenotype. However, not all exons can be removed while preserving C7 functionality, so this approach is not suitable for all mutations [19, 20]. Moreover, although efficient, the NHEJ-mediated method produces a heterogenous mixture of gene products through indel mutations, which can create clinical safety concerns.

Dominant dystrophic EB (DDEB) has dominant negative pathogenicity, as C7 production from the mutated allele impairs the gene product from the normal allele. NHEJ CRISPR/Cas9 can induce nonsense mutations in the mutated allele, resulting in rapid degradation of pathogenic RNA and protein, leaving normal C7 protein unimpaired. Shinkuma et al. demonstrated this in iPSCs for treating a causative DDEB mutation in exon 109 of C7 [14]. The study importantly validated that the CRISPR-Cas9 system was sufficiently specific to not target the unmutated allele and suggests that similar approaches can be adopted for other dominant negative genodermatoses, such as EBS.

HDR-dependent CRISPR-Cas9 approaches have been pursued for other mutations in EB. Izmiryan and colleagues edited an RDEB mutation and, notably, did not employ antibiotic or fluorescence-based selection for edited clones, which is a key step toward clinical applicability [21]. Low HDR efficiency in primary patient cells resulted in a correction rate of 15.7% [22, 23]. Murine grafting demonstrated that the 26% C7 rescue in this study was sufficient to form AFs; however, the minimum levels of C7 required to maintain skin stability are cited elsewhere to be 35%, suggesting the efficiency of this method may not be sufficient to promote full AF formation in RDEB patients [24].

The low efficiency (0.5%–20%) of HDR in post-mitotic cells is because HDR is only active after DNA replication in dividing cells [1]. To solve this, proliferative induced pluripotent stem cells (iPSCs) can be derived from primary cells to facilitate efficient HDR-based editing and isolation of edited single cell clones [25, 26]. Jackòw et al demonstrated the feasibility of this pipeline by using CRISPR-Cas9 to target *COL7A1* mutations in RDEB patient–derived iPSCs [27]. They successfully corrected monoallelic and biallelic mutations at an efficiency of up to 58% and 42%, respectively, and directed differentiation of edited iPSCs into 3-D human skin equivalents (HSEs). Grafting of HSEs onto mice evoked C7 deposition and AF formation, reversing the hallmark of the RDEB phenotype. Although patient-derived iPSCs can increase editing efficiency and circumvent the low expansion tolerance of primary cells, iPSCs have limitations [27]. Generation of iPSCs without immunogenic animal-derived products is not yet fully established for clinical applications. Rapid proliferation can also result in mutation acquisition in oncogenes and tumor suppressors such as p53, increasing the risk of tumors upon *in vivo* implantation [28, 29]. Xeno-free iPSC protocols and rigorous genomic integrity testing are therefore clearly essential for the future of iPSCs in clinical pipelines for Genodermatoses [30]. Low-efficiency HDR can also be ameliorated through NHEJ inhibitors, commercial HDR enhancer reagents, and chemically modified DNA donor templates, which, collectively, can increase HDR rates up to seven-fold [31].

The potential of CRISPR-Cas9 is evident; however, safety concerns remain [32]. Cas9 may cleave off-target sites on the genome with similar sequences to the target, introducing unwanted DSBs and mutations [33] and creating potentially deleterious effects on gene function or tumorigenicity. It is therefore warranted to mitigate off-target editing in any clinical gene editing tool. This can be countered by careful design of gRNAs using *in silico* tools such as the CRISPR Design Tool (Broad Institute) [33] and genome-wide off-target screening after editing [34]. The development of highly specific nucleases, such as high-fidelity Cas9 [Cas9-HF1], can also lead to almost undetectable off-target editing [32]. Furthermore, an innovative strategy has used a modified Cas9 effector, known as Cas9 nickase (Cas9n), to diminish off-target effects when correcting an RDEB mutation [35]. Cas9n creates "nicks," or single-strand breaks, at a target site, but it can be used with two gRNAs to create a "double-nicking" effect on each strand and a staggered "DSB" at the target locus. This was shown to improve not only the off-target safety profile but also the HDR efficiency [35].

In addition to the described therapeutic strategies, CRISPR-Cas9 can be harnessed as a tool for disease modeling of genodermatoses. Netherton syndrome (NS) is a recessive condition characterised by a non-functional skin barrier, icthyosiform keratoderma, bamboo-like hair, and atopic diathesis [36] and is caused by mutations in *SPINK5* encoding the LEKTI protein. A group generated faithful *in vitro* and *in vivo* models of NS by targeting *SPINK5* to excise exon 1 by NHEJ in human keratinocytes, with up to 81% of alleles carrying the deletion [37]. Impressively, NS constructs then treated by *ex vivo* lentiviral gene transfer of *SPINK5* showed recovery of LEKTI expression and normalization of the epidermal architecture on *in vivo* xeno-grafts. This proved the concept of using CRISPR-Cas9 to develop a disease-modeling and human cell–based testing platform for therapies for NS and other genodermatoses.

Base Editing

Base Editing is a novel gene editing tool that can precisely install point mutations in a sequence without donor DNA templates or DSBs [38]. Due to this, products of base editing have minimal indel formation compared to

CRISPR-Cas9 and other gene editing tools[39]. Also, as precise editing does not rely on the incorporation of a donor template via HDR, far higher efficiencies of gene correction can be achieved, especially in post-mitotic cells [40, 41]. Base editors were developed by fusing a catalytically impaired Cas9 nuclease (dCas9) to a single stranded DNA-specific cytidine deaminase enzyme [42]. dCas9 can bind to specific genomic sequences using a gRNA; however, it cannot cleave the DNA backbone once bound [40]. Instead, dCas9 exposes a short section of the genomic DNA into a single-stranded "R-loop," which provides a substrate for the cytidine deaminase enzyme to modify the DNA [39]. Cytidine deaminase converts cytosine bases into uridine, which is read as a tyrosine, thereby effecting a permanent C > T substitution [40] and creating a subsequent G > A change on the complementary strand. Base editing was augmented by replacing cytidine deaminase with an adenine deaminase enzyme to yield a class of "adenine base editors" (ABEs) that can convert A•T base pairs to G•C pairs [43]. Together, the advent of cytosine base editors (CBEs) and ABEs facilitate the programmable introduction of all four transitions (C > T, A > G, T > C and G > A) in the genome [43].

A majority of known single base pair pathogenic mutations are reported to be transition SNPs, which are possible to correct by base editing [44]. Nonsense mutations occur when arginine, encoded by CGA, is changed into a premature termination codon (TGA), and this often leads to nonsense-mediated decay of truncated mRNA and severe phenotypes due to total absence of protein expression. These recurrent C > T mutations in skin disease are possible to reverse using ABE [41]. Contrarily, CBEs can mutate trinucleotides into stop codons [45], which is a promising strategy to precisely disrupt genes for disease modeling and therapeutic knock out of mutant alleles in dominant negative conditions.

These advantages have positioned base editing as a highly attractive option; however, current impediments to their therapeutic application have also emerged. Akin to Cas9 nucleases, base editors require a 5'-NGG protospacer adjacent motif (PAM) sequence to be sited downstream of the target site to bind. In contrast, the reliance of an R loop to form strictly limits the editing of canonical ABEs and CBEs to nucleotides within an "activity window" at positions 4 through 8 upstream of a PAM sequence at positions 21 through 23 [46]. This exquisite specificity means that approximately 74% of pathogenic transition mutations were not targetable by canonical base editing due to an inappropriately placed PAM site [47]. Nonetheless, work has since broadened the scope of base editors by expanding activity windows and also altering the dCas9 nuclease to recognize alternative PAM sites [39].

Although they confer less genome-wide off-target editing than CRISPR-Cas9, a further limitation is that CBEs and ABEs can cause undesired off-target changes to other cytosines or adenines, respectively, in the activity window. This so-called "bystander editing" is more prevalent with an expanded activity window, and therefore, a careful balance between targeting scope and off-target tendency must be considered when selecting a base editor variant. For therapeutic use, minimal bystander edits are essential, and this can be achieved by selecting variants that have narrowed activity windows and high sequence context specificity [39]. A suite of base editors has now been engineered that show greatly reduced bystander editing compared to preexisting variants, while retaining robust on-target effects [48]. The base editor eA3A-BE3 has lower bystander editing by only efficiently targeting cytidines that follow a thymine, correcting a human β-thalassemia mutation with 40-fold higher degree of precision [47].

The continuous advances of base editing into a safer and more effective tool bodes well for its future therapeutic use in genodermatoses. However, there is currently a paucity of data investigating its potential. Osborn and coworkers employed ABE to correct *ex vivo* COL7A1 mutations in RDEB fibroblasts and achieved correction rates of 23.8% and 8.2% for homozygous and heterozygous mutations [41]. Full-length C7 expression was rescued and demonstrated *in vitro* and *in vivo* mice tissue. There was, however, detectable bystander editing and, although it led to conservative Val > Ala amino acid changes, these can still be a concern for therapeutic application. This highlights the importance of selecting an activity window and base editor variants to minimize bystander editing.

An optimised variant of ABE, known as "ABE8" has been developed since the "ABEmax" version used by Osborn and coworkers [41, 49]. ABE8 further enhances the efficiency of ABEs and edited CD34+ cells at a rate of 60% and primary human T cells up to 99% [50]. Chemical modifications to stabilize the mRNA encoding an ABE and its gRNA have also mediated more efficient editing [51]. Strides have optimized the efficiency of CBEs for targeting a variety of mammalian cell types [52].

In the fast-evolving field of base editing, other promising advancements are on the horizon, including "CG" base editors (CGBE), which can convert C•G into G•C base pairs, facilitating the correction of transversion mutations by base editing for the first time [53]. It is worth noting, however, that the mechanism of base editing limits it to correcting substitution mutations only. Other tools need to be harnessed to target pathogenic insertions and deletions. Nevertheless, it is clear that base editing can have an ever-increasing role in the future study and therapy of genodermatoses.

Prime Editing

Liu and coworkers, the same team that developed base editing, recently described an entirely new method of genome editing known as "prime editing" [54].

Prime editing pioneers a DSB-free strategy of introducing targeted insertions, deletions, and all base substitutions. Prime editing utilises a prime editing guide RNA (pegRNA), which directs a Cas9 nickase to the desired target site, generating a single-strand break, or "nick," in the PAM-containing strand. The pegRNA also encodes an edited sequence, and this hybridizes to the cut strand, leaving an exposed 3'-hydroxyl group. This group primes the reverse transcription of an extension to this end which creates a 3' flap containing the edit. The unedited 5' flap can be excised by endogenous endonucleases, such as FEN1 and EXO1, driving the inclusion of the edited DNA into the heteroduplex. Finally, cell-mediated DNA repair of the unedited strand results in a permanent edit. Prime editor strategies therefore typically include two components: a pegRNA and a prime editor (PE) protein containing an RNA-guided DNA-nicking domain tethered to a reverse transcriptase (RT) domain.

Prime editor 3 (PE3) is the latest PE variant and differs from prime editor 2 (PE2) by inducing an additional single-strand break on the non-edited strand to promote greater cell-mediated repair [55]. PE3 thereby achieves efficiencies three-fold higher than PE2 and has demonstrated the introduction of 12 combinations of insertions, deletions, and/or point mutations across three genomic loci at an average editing rate of 55%. PE3 has editing efficiencies comparable to CRISPR-Cas9 mediated HDR while attaining a significantly lower rate of indel mutations and off-target editing. Prime editors have also been assessed alongside base editors. BE4max, a newer CBE variant, delivered higher editing efficiencies than PE3; however, it also created several bystander edits that PE3 did not. The indel frequency for both strategies was equally low.

Prime editors have shown early promise for the correction of sickle cell and Tay-Sachs disease mutations with high efficiency and minimal undesired effects. Thus far, there have been no reported studies examining its role for genodermatoses, although this will soon change.

UNFINISHED BUSINESS

The delivery of gene editing tools to target patient cells remains a significant hurdle in bridging the gap between preclinical studies and the bedside. The commonality between all gene editing technologies mentioned previously is that they require a method to efficiently enter target cells to effect therapeutic changes on the genome (Figure 9.1). Current strategies can be broadly categorized into two main classes: *ex vivo* and *in vivo* delivery [56].

Ex vivo strategies involve editing autologous cells removed from the patient, or cells derived from other sources, in the laboratory setting. Gene-edited cells are then transplanted back to the patient by injection or grafting. During *ex vivo* delivery, electroporation can permeate cells with the nucleic acid or ribonucleoprotein (RNP) form of gene editors while delivery using viral vectors or lipid nanoparticles has also been described [56]. Viral vectors have the disadvantage of permitting continuous expression of nucleases, whereas mRNA and protein delivery via electroporation allows transient editing activity, which reduces off-target effects. *Ex vivo* approaches currently have higher editing rates than *in vivo* systems and allow quality control of editing outcomes before transplantation; however, there are no clinical *ex vivo* studies yet for genodermatoses. *Ex vivo* remains the strategy of choice for most other gene editing clinical trials, the most advanced of which are in cancer immunotherapy and haemoglobinopathies [57]. In dermatology, *ex vivo* gene addition therapy has been pioneered clinically, using epidermal sheet transplantation and fibroblast injections, suggesting similar approaches could be adopted for future gene editing cell therapies [12, 13, 58]. However, the significant site-specific heterogeneity of the skin combined with its large surface area can pose a challenge for global *ex vivo* treatment [59].

In vivo systems, in which direct genome editing occurs *in situ* on a patient, could allow the targeting of multiple tissues simultaneously and is therefore clinically relevant in genodermatoses that have systemic manifestation or a large region to treat. Furthermore, *in vivo* editing can exert therapeutic benefits on cells that cannot be easily cultured and corrected *ex vivo* and those that do not travel back to their tissue of origin after transplantation. However, as cells cannot be screened for adverse editing during *in vivo* therapy, the required threshold for biosafety is greater and demands further optimization of gene editors.

Investigated routes of *in vivo* delivery include viral, lipid nanoparticles, cell-penetrating peptides (CPP), and nanomaterials [53]. Of the viral vectors, adeno-associated viruses (AAV) have perhaps the most promise due to their lower immunogenicity and lack of genome integration. However, the maximum AAV packaging size limits the delivery of whole editors, meaning the components may need to be split. Lipid nanoparticles, on the other hand, allow the delivery of whole ready-assembled RNP complexes and so facilitate rapid responses and controlled dosing, which minimizes off-target editing. Strikingly, they have been shown to administer Cas9 to the cells of rats *in vivo* with 97% knockdown efficiency [60]. However, its immunogenic profile in humans must still be fully characterized. CPPs have also shown early promise for shuttling Cas9 RNPs [61]. However, their toxicity and immunogenicity are yet to be fully explored, and, as is the case with gold and polymer nanoparticles, they have not yet shown efficacy with base editors [53]. Exosomes are naturally occurring extracellular vehicles (EVs) that can bind with cell membranes and secrete CRISPR Cas9 RNP complexes intracellularly following *in vivo* injection [62]. Further work to reduce their potential cell toxicity may result in a robust delivery system for large genome editing cargos.

SUMMARY

The CRISPR-Cas9 gene editing system has revolutionized the field through robust editing of a range of mutations and cell lines, precise targeting, and the simplicity of designing new gRNAs. Surmounting challenges relating to off-target editing, indel formation, and low HDR efficiency can provide an imminent future role for clinical use in genodermatoses.

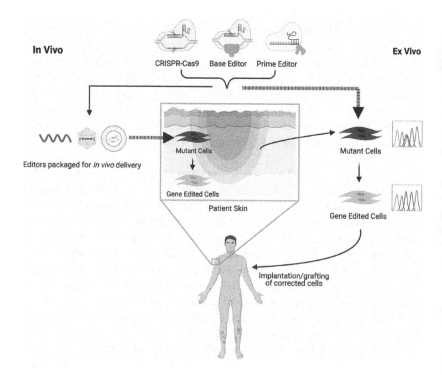

FIGURE 9.1 An overview of current gene editing strategies for genodermatoses, including CRISPR-Cas9, base editors and prime editors. *Ex vivo* and *in vivo* delivery methods are also shown. (Created with BioRender.com.)

Base editors and prime editors may offer synergistic capabilities. Base editors can efficiently correct transition mutations when no or few bystander bases are within the activity window. Alternatively, prime editors can correct insertions, deletions, and transversions when bystander base editing is likely, or the target nucleotide is not in an activity window. Data on the effectiveness of prime editing in different cell lines and its genome-wide off-target profile still remain to be examined and will be paramount in assessing its future scope.

Alongside expanding the gene editing toolbox, work has better established both *ex vivo* and *in vivo* delivery strategies for CRISPR-Cas9, base editor, and prime editor systems.

Therefore, despite being considered an impossibility, major strides in gene editing have now enabled the "scarless," targeted correction of all pathogenic mutations in genodermatoses to be on the horizon. Challenges remain relating to off-target editing, inconsistent efficiency, and delivery strategies, particularly for *in vivo* use. However, in the words of the double Nobel laureate Marie Curie, it is often the case that "One never notices what has been done; one can only see what remains to be done." This chapter aimed to outline how breakthroughs have led to an explosion in translational studies achieving promising progress. The first clinical trials for gene editing in genodermatoses will undoubtably occur soon and pave the way for an exciting future for researchers, clinicians, and patients.

REFERENCES

1. Guitart JR, Johnson JL, and Chien WW. Research techniques made simple: The application of CRISPR-Cas9 and genome editing in investigative dermatology. *J. Invest. Dermatol.* Elsevier B.V. 2016; 136.
2. Li H, Yang Y, Hong W, et al. Applications of genome editing technology in the targeted therapy of human diseases: Mechanisms, advances and prospects. *Signal Transduct. Target. Ther.* Springer Nature 2020; 5.
3. Bonafont J, Mencía Á, García M, et al. Clinically relevant correction of recessive dystrophic epidermolysis bullosa by dual sgRNA CRISPR/Cas9-mediated gene editing. *Mol. Ther* 2019; 27: 986–998.
4. Moreno AM and Mali P. Therapeutic genome engineering via CRISPR-Cas systems. *Wiley Interdiscip. Rev. Syst. Biol. Med* 2017; 9: e1380.
5. Jeong YK, Song B, and Bae S. Current status and challenges of DNA base editing tools. *Mol. Ther.* Cell Press 2020; 28.
6. Baker C and Hayden MS. Gene editing in dermatology: Harnessing CRISPR for the treatment of cutaneous disease. *F1000Research* 2020; 9: 281.

7. Salam A, Proudfoot LE, and McGrath JA. Inherited blistering skin diseases: Underlying molecular mechanisms and emerging therapies. *Ann. Med* 2014; 46: 49–61.

8. Has C, South A, and Uitto J. Molecular therapeutics in development for epidermolysis bullosa: Update 2020. *Mol. Diagn. Ther.* Adis 2020; 24).

9. Naso G and Petrova A. CRISPR/Cas9 gene editing for genodermatoses: Progress and perspectives. *Emerg. Top. Life Sci.* Portland Press Ltd 2019; 3.

10. Mavilio F, Pellegrini G, Ferrari S, et al. Correction of junctional epidermolysis bullosa by transplantation of genetically modified epidermal stem cells. *Nat. Med* 2006; 12: 1397–1402.

11. De Rosa L, Carulli S, Cocchiarella F, et al. Long-term stability and safety of transgenic cultured epidermal stem cells in gene therapy of junctional epidermolysis bullosa. *Stem Cell Rep* 2014; 2: 1–8.

12. Hirsch T, Rothoeft T, Teig N, et al. Regeneration of the entire human epidermis using transgenic stem cells. *Nature* 2017; 551: 327–332.

13. Siprashvili Z, Nguyen NT, Gorell ES, et al. Safety and wound outcomes following genetically corrected autologous epidermal grafts in patients with recessive dystrophic epidermolysis bullosa. *JAMA—J. Am. Med. Assoc* 2016; 316: 1808–1817.

14. Shinkuma S, Guo Z, and Christiano AM. Site-specific genome editing for correction of induced pluripotent stem cells derived from dominant dystrophic epidermolysis bullosa. *Proc. Natl. Acad. Sci. U. S. A* 2016; 113: 5676–5681.

15. Benati D, Miselli F, Cocchiarella F, et al. CRISPR/Cas9-mediated in situ correction of LAMB3 gene in keratinocytes derived from a junctional epidermolysis bullosa patient. *Mol. Ther* 2018; 26: 2592–2603.

16. Jinek M, Chylinski K, Fonfara I, et al. A programmable dual-RNA—guided DNA endonuclease in adaptive bacterial immunity. *Science* 2012; 337: 816–821.

17. Cong L, Ran FA, Cox D, et al. Multiplex genome engineering using CRISPR/Cas systems. *Science* 2013; 339: 819–823.

18. Mali P, Yang L, Esvelt KM, et al. RNA-guided human genome engineering via Cas9. *Science* 2013; 339: 823–826.

19. Bornert O, Kühl T, Bremer J, et al. Analysis of the functional consequences of targeted exon deletion in COL7A1 reveals prospects for dystrophic epidermolysis bullosa therapy. *Mol. Ther* 2016; 24(7): 1302–1311.

20. Turczynski S, Titeux M, Tonasso L, et al. Targeted exon skipping restores type VII collagen expression and anchoring fibril formation in an in vivo RDEB model. *J. Invest. Dermatol* 2016; 136(12): 2387–2395.

21. Izmiryan A, Ganier C, Bovolenta M, et al. Ex Vivo COL7A1 correction for recessive dystrophic epidermolysis bullosa using CRISPR/Cas9 and homology-directed repair. *Mol. Ther—Nucleic Acids* 2018; 12: 554–567.

22. Izmiryan A, Danos O, and Hovnanian A. Meganuclease-mediated COL7A1 gene correction for recessive dystrophic epidermolysis bullosa. *J. Invest. Dermatol* 2016; 136(4): 872–875.

23. Osborn MJ, Starker CG, McElroy AN, et al. TALEN-based gene correction for epidermolysis bullosa. *Mol. Ther* 2013; 21: 1151–1159.

24. Tolar J and Wagner JE. Allogeneic blood and bone marrow cells for the treatment of severe epidermolysis bullosa: Repair of the extracellular matrix. *The Lancet* 2013; 382(9899): 1214–1223.

25. Yumlu S, Stumm J, Bashir S, et al. Gene editing and clonal isolation of human induced pluripotent stem cells using CRISPR/Cas9. *Methods* 2017; 121–122: 29–44.

26. Takahashi K, Tanabe K, Ohnuki M, et al. Induction of pluripotent stem cells from adult human fibroblasts by defined factors. *Cell* 2007; 131(5): 861–872.

27. Jacków J, Guo Z, Hansen C, et al. CRISPR/Cas9-based targeted genome editing for correction of recessive dystrophic epidermolysis bullosa using iPS cells. *Proc. Natl. Acad. Sci. U. S. A* 2019; 116: 26846–26852.

28. Ihry RJ, Worringer KA, Salick MR, et al. P53 inhibits CRISPR-Cas9 engineering in human pluripotent stem cells. *Nat. Med* 2018; 24: 939–946.

29. Lee AS, Tang C, Rao MS, et al. Tumorigenicity as a clinical hurdle for pluripotent stem cell therapies. *Nat. Med* 2013; 19: 998–1004.

30. Jeriha J, Kolundzic N, Khurana P, et al. mRNA-based reprogramming under xeno-free and feeder-free conditions. *Methods Mol. Biol. Clifton NJ* 2020.

31. Skarnes WC, Pellegrino E, and McDonough JA. Improving homology-directed repair efficiency in human stem cells. *Methods* 2019; 164–165: 18–28.

32. Uitto J, Bruckner-Tuderman L, Christiano AM, et al. Progress toward treatment and cure of epidermolysis bullosa: Summary of the DEBRA international research symposium EB2015. *J. Invest. Dermatol.* Elsevier B.V. 2016; 136.

33. Ran FA, Hsu PD, Wright J, et al. Genome engineering using the CRISPR-Cas9 system. *Nat. Protoc* 2013; 8: 2281–2308.

34. Khan SH. Genome-editing technologies: Concept, pros, and cons of various genome-editing techniques and bioethical concerns for clinical application. *Mol. Ther—Nucleic Acids.* Cell Press 2019; 16.

35. Kocher T, Wagner RN, Klausegger A, et al. Improved double-nicking strategies for COL7A1-editing by homologous recombination. *Mol. Ther—Nucleic Acids* 2019; 18: 496–507.

36. Hannula-Jouppi K, Laasanen SL, Ilander M. et al. Intrafamily and interfamilial phenotype variation and immature immunity in patients with Netherton syndrome and Finnish SPINK5 founder mutation. *JAMA Dermatol* 2016; 152(4): 435–442.

37. Gálvez V, Chacón-Solano E, Bonafont J, et al. Efficient CRISPR-Cas9-mediated gene ablation in human keratinocytes to recapitulate genodermatoses: Modeling of Netherton syndrome. *Mol. Ther-Methods Clin. Dev* 2020; 18: 280–290.

38. Anzalone AV, Koblan LW, and Liu DR. Genome editing with CRISPR—Cas nucleases, base editors, transposases and prime editors. *Nat. Biotechnol.* Nature Research 2020; 38.

39. Huang TP, Newby GA, and Liu DR. Precision genome editing using cytosine and adenine base editors in mammalian cells. *Nat. Protoc* 2021; 16: 1089–1128.

40. Komor AC, Kim YB, Packer MS, et al. Programmable editing of a target base in genomic DNA without double-stranded DNA cleavage. *Nature* 2016; 533: 420–424.

41. Osborn MJ, Newby GA, McElroy AN, et al. Base editor correction of COL7A1 in recessive dystrophic epidermolysis bullosa patient-derived fibroblasts and iPSCs. *J. Invest. Dermatol* 2020; 140: 338–347.e5.

42. Komor AC, Badran AH, and Liu DR. Editing the genome without double-stranded DNA breaks. *ACS Chem. Biol.* American Chemical Society 2018; 13.

43. Gaudelli NM, Komor AC, Rees HA, et al. Programmable base editing of T to G C in genomic DNA without DNA cleavage. *Nature* 2017; 551: 464–471.

44. Whittock NV, Ashton GHS, Mohammedi R, et al. Comparative mutation detection screening of the type VII collagen gene (COL7A1) using the protein truncation test, fluorescent chemical cleavage of mismatch, and conformation sensitive gel electrophoresis. *J. Invest. Dermatol* 1999; 113(4): 673–686.

45. Rees HA and Liu DR. Base editing: Precision chemistry on the genome and transcriptome of living cells. *Nat. Rev. Genet.* Nature Publishing Group 2018; 19.

46. Coluccio A, Miselli F, Lombardo A, et al. Targeted gene addition in human epithelial stem cells by zinc-finger nuclease-mediated homologous recombination. *Mol. Ther* 2013; 21: 1695–1704.

47. Gehrke JM, Cervantes O, Clement MK, et al. An APOBEC3A-Cas9 base editor with minimized bystander and off-target activities. *Nat. Biotechnol* 2018; 36: 977–982.

48. Doman JL, Raguram A, Newby GA. et al. Evaluation and minimization of Cas9-independent off-target DNA editing by cytosine base editors. *Nat. Biotechnol* 2020; 38(5): 620–628.

49. Richter MF, Zhao KT, Eton E. et al. Phage-assisted evolution of an adenine base editor with improved Cas domain compatibility and activity. *Nat. Biotechnol* 2020; 38: 883–891.

50. Gaudelli NM, Lam DK, Rees HA, et al. Directed evolution of adenine base editors with increased activity and therapeutic application. *Nat. Biotechnol* 2020; 38: 892–900.

51. Jiang T, Henderson JM, Coote K, et al. Chemical modifications of adenine base editor mRNA and guide RNA expand its application scope. *Nat. Commun* 2020; 11: 1979.

52. Koblan LW, Doman JL, Wilson C, et al. Improving cytidine and adenine base editors by expression optimization and ancestral reconstruction. *Nat. Biotechnol* 2018; 36: 843–846.

53. Porto EM, Komor AC, Slaymaker IM, et al. Base editing: Advances and therapeutic opportunities. *Nat. Rev. Drug Discov* 2020; 19: 839–859.

54. Anzalone AV, Randolph PB, Davis JR, et al. Search-and-replace genome editing without double-strand breaks or donor DNA. *Nature* 2019: 576; 149–157.

55. Matsoukas IG. Prime editing: Genome editing for rare genetic diseases without double-strand breaks or donor DNA. *Front. Genet* 2020: 11.

56. Cox DBT, Platt RJ, and Zhang F. Therapeutic genome editing: Prospects and challenges. *Nat. Med* 2015; 21: 121–131.

57. Ernst MPT, Broeders M, Herrero-Hernandez P, et al. Ready for repair? Gene editing enters the clinic for the treatment of human disease. *Mol. Ther—Methods Clin. Dev.* Cell Press 2020; 18.

58. Lwin SM, Syed F, Di WL, et al. Safety and early efficacy outcomes for lentiviral fibroblast gene therapy in recessive dystrophic epidermolysis bullosa. *JCI Insight* 2019; 4.

59. Sriram G, Bigliardi PL, and Bigliardi-Qi M. Fibroblast heterogeneity and its implications for engineering organotypic skin models in vitro. *Eur. J. Cell Biol.* Elsevier GmbH 2015; 94.

60. Itoh M, Kawagoe S, Tamai K, et al. Footprint-free gene mutation correction in induced pluripotent stem cell (iPSC) derived from recessive dystrophic epidermolysis bullosa (RDEB) using the CRISPR/Cas9 and piggyBac transposon system. *J. Dermatol. Sci* 2020; 98: 163–172.

61. Krishnamurthy S, Wohlford-Lenane C, Kandimalla S, et al. Engineered amphiphilic peptides enable delivery of proteins and CRISPR-associated nucleases to airway epithelia. *Nat. Commun* 2019; 10: 4906.

62. Gee P, Lung MSY, Okuzaki Y, et al. Extracellular nanovesicles for packaging of CRISPR-Cas9 protein and sgRNA to induce therapeutic exon skipping. *Nat. Commun* 2020; 11: 1334.

Ex vivo Gene Therapy for Epidermolysis Bullosa

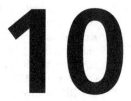

10

Işın Sinem Bağcı, Kunju Sridhar, John A. M. Dolorito, and M. Peter Marinkovich

Contents

INTRODUCTION

Epidermolysis bullosa (EB) is a family of genetically inherited skin disorders that is characterized by weakened skin integrity and that share the common trait of blistering in response to external mechanical trauma. The EB group

DOI: 10.1201/9781003121275-14

of diseases are a classic example of genes and the environment interacting together to drive disease pathology. EB was first clinically recognized over 150 years ago [1], and the three major subtypes—EB simplex, junctional EB, and dystrophic EB—were recognized a hundred years ago. Since that time, it has been a long journey to build the foundation of knowledge we currently have about the clinical EB variants and their underlying molecular pathologies [2]. It is only through this foundation of knowledge, built over the years, that genetic therapies for EB have finally been developed. This chapter examines our first successful clinical trials of gene therapy for this group of diseases. It has been the case that skin, being such an accessible organ, has led the way in gene therapy research, and much of what we have learned from cutaneous gene therapy for EB provides valuable information to help guide future gene therapy for other diseases affecting less accessible extracutaneous tissues.

Through the course of evolution, beginning with amphibians and progressing through mammalian species, a specialized basement membrane structure has evolved at the interface of epithelial and mesenchymal tissues. This evolutionary enhancement, termed the anchoring complex [3], was first visualized by transmission electron microscopy as a specialized ultrastructural entity in those tissues exposed to the external environment such as the eyes; the nasopharyngeal, oropharyngeal and laryngotracheal mucosa; the bladder and distal genitourinary tract; the proximal and distal gastrointestinal tract; and, most especially, the skin [4, 5]. In time, the proteins that make up the anchoring complex were biochemically characterized, their cellular origins were determined [6, 7], and it was appreciated that these proteins evolved with the purpose of providing added tissue cohesion in the face of disruptive external forces. Underlying gene mutations causing defects in two of the most critical anchoring complex components, laminin-332 and collagen VII, represent the molecular basis for most cases of junctional epidermolysis bullosa (JEB) and all cases of dystrophic epidermolysis bullosa (DEB), respectively [8].

Laminin-332 is a critical epithelial adhesive protein containing $\alpha3$, $\beta3$, and $\gamma2$ subunits [9]. Laminin-332 promotes tissue integrity by complexing with other laminins to form ultrastructural entities termed anchoring filaments [10]. Laminin-332 is normally present in skin and oropharyngeal and laryngeal basement membranes; however, it is absent in tissues affected by severe-JEB [11]. It is well established that laminin-332 deficiency is the cause of most cases of JEB [12, 13]. Type VII collagen is a large, triple-helical-shaped protein including 8,833 nucleotides [14]. It consists of a central collagenous triple-helical domain flanked by two noncollagenous domains, NC1 and NC2 [6]. While the NC1 domain interacts with fibronectin, laminin 332, type I, and type IV collagen to provide dermal-epidermal attachment [15, 16], the NC2 domain initiates the triple-helical assembly of type VII collagen [17].

ANALYSIS OF THE NEED

JEB has the most heterogenous underlying gene defects, affecting gene coding for one of several basement membrane proteins, including collagen XVII, α6β4 integrin, and plectin. However, the majority of JEB cases are caused by mutations of genes coding for laminin-332, in particular the LAMB3 gene coding for the β3 subunit of laminin-332. True null mutations of laminin-332 genes result in Severe-JEB, which affects a fifth of all JEB patients. Severe-JEB is extremely lethal [8], with 90% of patients dying in the first year of life [18]. According to an extensive survey, the average age of death was 5.8 months, with the four most common causes of death being failure to thrive, respiratory failure, pneumonia, and dehydration [19]. Overall, the findings suggest that while cutaneous blistering is severe, it is the mucosal erosions that lead to lethal complications. These mucosal complications include oral erosions, which impair feeding, leading to weight loss, dehydration, and failure to thrive. Other, just as serious mucosal complications include laryngotracheal erosions, which cause airway obstruction [20], leading to dyspnea, stridor, pneumonia, and respiratory arrest (Orphanet online database, orpha.net, entry Orpha:79404). Currently, no corrective therapy exists for Severe-JEB. Once diagnosed, therapy consists of comfort care to ease suffering until the patient dies [18, 19]. Less severe laminin-332 gene mutations resulting in only a partial loss of laminin-332 function can produce a non-lethal but still severe form termed intermediate JEB with less severe mucosal disease or a still milder form termed localized JEB with limited skin blistering [2, 21].

Based on recent genomic modeling studies, recessive dystrophic epidermolysis bullosa (RDEB) has an estimated incidence of 95 per million live births, and it is estimated to affect nearly 4,000 patients in the United States [22]. RDEB is associated with deleterious mutations in *COL7A1* gene encoding type VII collagen [23]. Type VII collagen is synthesized by both keratinocytes and fibroblasts to form anchoring fibrils (AFs), which anchor the epidermis to the dermis [7]. Dysfunctional *COL7A1* gene and type VII collagen lead to a lack of dermal-epidermal adhesion, resulting in subepidermal blisters located at the sites of trauma; mutilating scarring, including fusion of fingers (pseudosyndactyly); esophageal stenosis; and joint contractures, as well as absent or deformed nails and malformed teeth [2]. In addition, severe RDEB patients show an ultimately shortened life span, with a 70% risk of death by age 45 due to aggressive metastatic SCC development arising within chronic wounds [24]. Milder RDEB variants, including intermediate, inversa, and localized RDEB subtypes, also are caused by less function-disrupting *COL7A1* mutations [21].

THE TECHNOLOGY: *EX VIVO* GENE THERAPY

Ex vivo Gene Therapy in Junctional Epidermolysis Bullosa

Recent gene therapy studies of non-lethal JEB patients have shown promising results. In the several patients studied, laminin-332 gene corrected cutaneous epidermal autografts have demonstrated remarkable take and persistence, with one patient showing over 80% of the entire gene-edited cutaneous surface with long-term correction [25, 26]. These studies were performed with the use of a modified *LAMB3* containing retroviral vector. Integrative viral mediated gene transfer, such as retroviral gene transfer, shows durable expression due to viral insertion of the therapeutic gene into the chromosome.

A key factor in the success of laminin-332 gene replacement lies in the absolute dependence of keratinocytes on laminin-332 expression for cell adhesion. Deprived of laminin-332 binding by introducing inhibitory laminin-332 antibodies into the culture medium, for example, normal keratinocytes round up and detach from the culture surface [27]. Similarly, laminin-332 deficient JEB keratinocytes show an inability to attach and require an adhesive coating on tissue culture plates; otherwise, they round up and fall off the culture surface [28]. This adhesive selection property is extremely useful following laminin-332 gene transfer as only transduced laminin-332 positive cells attach and grow, while non-adherent, non-transduced laminin-332 deficient cells are removed during *in vitro* cell expansion and graft production. Thus, this use of cell adhesion as an *in vitro* selection tool to generate pure cultures of laminin-332 expressing keratinocytes was undoubtedly a key factor in the success of laminin-332 epidermal autograft therapy for JEB [25].

The ability of laminin-332 inhibitory antibodies to detach epidermis from dermis in human and mouse skin suggests that laminin-332 plays a key role in supporting *in vivo* epithelial adhesion [27, 29]. This increased adhesive capacity would give transduced laminin-332 expressing JEB keratinocytes an ability to out compete and displace non-transduced laminin-332 negative epithelium. This would explain the observed expansion of corrected laminin-332 epidermis far outside of the original graft boundaries [25]. In addition, laminin-332 is an important promoter of keratinocyte stem cell growth and persistence [25, 30]. Together, these factors account for the high level of graft take and clinical improvement seen in JEB patients following laminin-332 gene therapy.

Ex vivo Gene Therapy in Recessive Dystrophic Epidermolysis Bullosa

Despite the technical difficulties of delivering a large-size gene such as full-length *COL7A1 (9kb)*, expression of type VII collagen (longer than two years) has been demonstrated on RDEB skin tissue regenerated on immunodeficient mice using Moloney leukemia virus–derived retroviral vector (LZRSE) [31]. Following this preclinical achievement, three RDEB patients with a mean age of 28.7 years have been treated with autologous keratinocyte sheets expressing full-length type VII collagen using LZRSE containing the *COL7A1* gene [32, 33]. Long-term follow-up reports demonstrated that ≥75% wound healing was achieved in 82%, 66%, 39%, 58%, and 70% of the treated wounds in the follow up periods of 3, 6, and 12 months; 2 years; and 3 years, respectively. Full-length type VII collagen expression on the treated areas was assessed via NC2 domain positivity, which was detected in 73% of biopsies (11 of 15) at 3 months, in 53% of biopsies (8 of 15) at 6 months, in 11% of biopsies (1 of 9) at 1 year, and 67% of biopsies (2 of 3) at 2 years. AFs were seen in 67% of biopsies (8 of 12) at 3 months, in 53% of biopsies (8 of 15) at 6 months, in 43% of biopsies (3 of 7) at 1 year, and 50% of biopsies (1 of 2) at 2 years. Significant wound healing response in concordance with durable recombinant type VII collagen expression in the engrafted tissues demonstrated by this study led to the phase 3 trial, which is currently ongoing (ClinicalTrials.gov identifier: NCT0422710).

However, this treatment also has limitations, such as the necessity of general anesthesia for grafting, various treatment responses in different anatomical sites (with decreased wound healing at back), and the grafts being not suitable for some problematic areas of RDEB patients (such as fingers and toes). In addition, the wound healing achieved in RDEB patients was maintained for a shorter time than in JEB patients treated with *LAMB3* engineered allogenic grafts [25, 26]. Analysis of holoclone stem cells in regenerated epidermis, which has been performed in JEB trials but not in RDEB trials, could be helpful to understand the underlying factors causing the difference in the longevity of RDEB and JEB wound healing [25].

Another factor that could affect the difference between the two trials might be the fact that, normally, *LAMB3* is expressed only by keratinocytes, whereas *COL7A1* is expressed by both keratinocytes and fibroblasts. Recently, it was reported that engineered skin substitutes produced type VII collagen in the presence of keratinocytes or fibroblasts; however, structurally normal AFs were seen only in the skin substitutes, including both keratinocytes and fibroblasts [34]. Although type VII collagen is mainly produced and secreted by epidermal keratinocytes and, to a lesser extent, by fibroblasts [7], gene transferred and grafted fibroblasts showed a higher ability of supplying type VII collagen to BMZ preclinically than gene transferred and grafted keratinocytes [35]. In addition, fibroblasts are more robust, can be cultured extensively, and are less susceptible to growth arrest and differentiation than keratinocytes [36], which makes them superior to keratinocytes for local wound treatment.

Following the preclinical demonstration of type VII collagen and AF restoration through intradermal injection of *COL7A1* transduced fibroblasts in immunodeficient xenograft mouse models [36, 37], the first human phase I study was conducted on four adult RDEB patients [38]. Lentiviral expressing *COL7A1*-modified autologous fibroblasts were intradermally injected over a 1 cm^2 area of intact skin. At month 12, two of the four subjects showed significant increase in type VII collagen expression as compared to control skin sites, although AF restoration was not detected in the treated areas [38]. Three of the four subjects had low baseline serum anti–type VII collagen IgG (by ELISA), which did not show significant changes throughout 12 months in two subjects. The third subject showed a two-fold increase at month 12; however, this serum showed no reaction in salt-split skin indirect immunofluorescence microscopy [38].

The second human phase I/II trial conducted by our group aimed to assess the therapeutic efficacy of gene-transferred autologous fibroblasts injection on persistent non-healing wounds of six RDEB patients (five adults, one child) throughout a follow up period of 52 weeks. Following the intradermal administration of Lentiviral-*COL7A1*-fibroblasts around the wounds, ≥75% wound healing was achieved in 70%, 80%, 75%, and 67% of the wounds at weeks 4, 12, 25, and 52, respectively. By contrast, ≥75% wound healing was observed in 10%, 11%, 0%, and 16% of untreated control wounds at weeks 4, 12, 25, and 52, respectively [39]. In addition, none of the subjects developed antibody response against type VII collagen [39]. Both of the human trials reported injection-related side effects, such as injection site erythema and discoloration, pain, etc., but no serious side effects that could be related to the gene-corrected fibroblasts. Taken together, *COL7A1*-modified autologous fibroblasts seem to be an effective and safe approach in the treatment of RDEB wounds. The phase III trial is currently ongoing (ClinicalTrials.gov identifier: NCT04213261).

THE UNFINISHED BUSINESS

Collagen VII gene therapy and laminin-332 gene therapy share their own strengths and weaknesses [40]. As for collagen VII gene therapy, it may not show the same selective adhesive advantages as laminin-332 gene therapy. For example, unlike laminin-332, collagen VII does not normally serve as a keratinocyte adhesion ligand, either *in vitro* or *in vivo*. Instead, keratinocytes only indirectly interact with collagen VII through collagen VII's association with laminin-332 [16]. As a result, collagen VII negative DEB keratinocytes show no *in vitro* attachment deficiencies [41]. Therefore, collagen VII positive DEB keratinocytes cannot be enriched by differential adhesion following COL7A1 transduction. This likely explains why collagen VII overexpressing epidermal autografts contain a substantial proportion (30%) of non-transduced cells [33], a phenomenon which dilutes the effectiveness of these epidermal autografts. There are no data to suggest collagen VII expression confers any selective *in vivo* adhesion advantage to transduced keratinocytes that could explain why collagen VII expressing epidermal grafts failed to expand beyond the graft borders and instead slowly declined over the year following placement onto recipient DEB patients [33].

Collagen VII gene therapy, on the other hand, has certain advantages. It is more widely applicable to a greater number of patients than laminin-332 gene therapy. For example, it can be used on the most severe or the milder variants of RDEB. In contrast, only non-lethal JEB patients and no severe-JEB patients have been treated with cutaneous laminin-332 gene therapy thus far [25, 26, 42]. This is because, even following cutaneous laminin-332 gene therapy, severe-JEB patients would still be expected to die from their severe mucosal disease. Thus, without any current technology to graft mucosal surfaces, cutaneous grafting of severe-JEB patients would be of little overall benefit.

Another advantage that collagen VII gene therapy has over laminin-332 gene therapy is in its theoretical potential for inducing immune reaction. Laminin-332 is an antigenic glycoprotein and a target in an autoimmune bullous skin disease [43, 44]. Patients with severe-JEB, with completely null expression of laminin-332, would be expected to have an immune system that does not recognize laminin-332 as self. Therapeutic introduction of laminin-332 expression would therefore be more likely, in theory, to induce an immune reaction. This has never been tested to date, as no laminin-332 null JEB patients have yet been treated. Instead, all of the patients treated with laminin-332 gene therapy had only missense mutations, usually with a single amino acid substitution. This type of patient selection helps avoid autoimmune reactions but would not benefit the majority of JEB patients, who have null mutation and severe disease.

In contrast, true null mutations occur in only 30% of severe RDEB patients and in none of the milder RDEB subvariants [45]. The majority of RDEB patients express at least the NC1 domain, which is known to be the most antigenic part of the type VII collagen molecule and which is the primary target of autoantibodies in epidermolysis bullosa acquisita [46]. It would be expected that RDEB patients who express NC1 domain would have a lesser chance of developing immune reactions to therapeutic type VII collagen, since the "new" part of type VII collagen would be the less antigenic one. In currently published reports, only NC1 positive RDEB patients have been treated so far, likely for this reason.

Despite this precaution however, two RDEB patients have developed tissue-bond antibodies against type VII collagen in response to gene therapy. One of them showed increased titer of anti-type VII collagen antibody (1:300) as compared to baseline value (1:40) directed against epitopes at or near the NC2 domain [33]. Taken that all subjects showed positive NC1 and negative NC2 at their baseline characteristics, an immune reaction against the recombinant type VII collagen seems to have occurred in this patient. From these experiences thus far, we should recognize that detecting and managing unwanted immune reactions to therapeutic gene products will be an important part of our gene therapy work in the future.

Another disadvantage of these *ex vivo* gene therapies is the integrative nature of therapeutic retroviral and lentiviral vectors. Since viral insertion by these vectors is random, it could modulate an oncogene or tumor suppressor gene, thereby influencing neoplasia development. This is more than a theoretical possibility, as illustrated by reported cases of development of leukemia in patients undergoing retroviral therapy for X-linked severe combined immuodeficiency disease [47, 48]. It is important to note that in the fibroblast RDEB studies mentioned earlier, *COL7A1* delivery was achieved by a lentiviral vector, which is accepted to be safer regarding the risk of insertional mutagenesis [49].

A new approach to *COL7A1* gene therapy using an episomal modified, replication defective, herpes simplex 1 vector applied topically directly to RDEB skin (in vivo gene therapy) could address this integrative oncogenesis safety concern. This new in vivo approach has several advantages in that it can be administered off the shelf without the need for cell engineering. Another advantage is that it is applied under basic outpatient conditions without the need for anesthesia or hospitalization (Figure 10.1), and therefore, it may be more accessible to greater numbers of patients, especially those patients in underdeveloped countries or without access to specialized medical centers. This trial of topical gene therapy is currently in a multisite phase III trial (ClinicalTrials.gov Identifier NCT04491604).

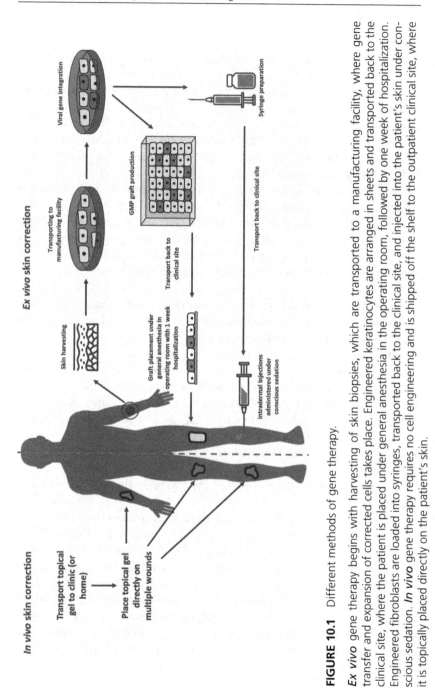

FIGURE 10.1 Different methods of gene therapy.

Ex vivo gene therapy begins with harvesting of skin biopsies, which are transported to a manufacturing facility, where gene transfer and expansion of corrected cells takes place. Engineered keratinocytes are arranged in sheets and transported back to the clinical site, where the patient is placed under general anesthesia in the operating room, followed by one week of hospitalization. Engineered fibroblasts are loaded into syringes, transported back to the clinical site, and injected into the patient's skin under conscious sedation. *In vivo* gene therapy requires no cell engineering and is shipped off the shelf to the outpatient clinical site, where it is topically placed directly on the patient's skin.

SUMMARY

A foundation of knowledge of the biology of the dermal-epidermal basement membrane and the pathophysiology of EB have paved the way for the first gene therapy clinical trials for JEB and RDEB. These trials have demonstrated proof of concept that gene therapy can be safely implemented, and they demonstrate durable correction of JEB and RDEB patient skin. A number of factors are needed to refine and enhance gene delivery to the skin. These include improvements in gene delivery, including refining *ex vivo* approaches, reducing the risk of cancer development by therapeutic vectors, better targeting of skin stem cells, development of new *in vivo* approaches, and preventing autoimmune reactions. These are the challenges that lie ahead for both gene therapy for epidermolysis bullosa and the gene therapy field as a whole.

REFERENCES

1. Hebra FV. Arztlicher Bericht des K.K allegemeinen Krankenhauses zu Wien vom Jare 1870. *Vienna* 1870; 362.
2. Bardhan A, Bruckner-Tuderman L, Chapple ILC, Fine J-D, Harper N, Has C, et al. Epidermolysis bullosa. *Nature Reviews Disease Primers* 2020; 6(1).
3. Ryan MC, Christiano AM, Engvall E, Wewer UM, Miner JH, Sanes JR, et al. The functions of laminins: Lessons from in vivo studies. *Matrix Biology Matrix Biol* 1996; 15(6): 369–381.
4. Palade GE and Farquhar MG. A special fibril of the dermis. *J Cell Biol* 1965; 27(1): 215–224.
5. Pearson RW. Studies on the pathogenesis of epidermolysis bullosa. *J Invest Dermatol* 1962; 39: 551–575.
6. Burgeson RE. Type VII collagen, anchoring fibrils, and epidermolysis bullosa. *J Invest Dermatol* 1993; 101(3): 252–255.
7. Marinkovich MP, Keene DR, Rimberg CS, Burgeson RE. Cellular origin of the dermal-epidermal basement membrane. *Dev Dyn* 1993; 197(4): 255–267.
8. Marinkovich MP. Inherited epidermolysis bullosa. In: Kang S, Amagai M, Bruckner AL, Enk AH, Margolis DJ, McMichael AJ, et al. Eds. *Fitzpatrick's Dermatology*. 9th Ed. McGraw-Hill Education, New York, NY, 2019; pp. 1011–1035.
9. Marinkovich MP, Lunstrum GP, and Burgeson RE. The anchoring filament protein kalinin is synthesized and secreted as a high molecular weight precursor. *J Biol Chem* 1992; 267(25): 17900–17906.
10. Marinkovich MP, Lunstrum GP, Keene DR, and Burgeson RE. The dermal-epidermal junction of human skin contains a novel laminin variant. *J Cell Biol* 1992; 119(3): 695–703.

11. Meneguzzi G, Marinkovich MP, Aberdam D, Pisani A, Burgeson R, and Ortonne JP. Kalinin is abnormally expressed in epithelial basement membranes of Herlitz's junctional epidermolysis bullosa patients. *Exp Dermatol* 1992; 1(5): 221–229.

12. Marinkovich MP, Meneguzzi G, Burgeson RE, Blanchet-Bardon C, Holbrook KA, Smith LT, et al. Prenatal diagnosis of Herlitz junctional epidermolysis bullosa by amniocentesis. *Prenat Diagn* 1995; 15(11): 1027–1034.

13. Marinkovich MP, Verrando P, Keene DR, Meneguzzi G, Lunstrum GP, Ortonne JP, et al. Basement membrane proteins kalinin and nicein are structurally and immunologically identical. *Lab Invest* 1993; 69(3): 295–299.

14. Christiano AM, Greenspan DS, Lee S, and Uitto J. Cloning of human type VII collagen. Complete primary sequence of the alpha 1(VII) chain and identification of intragenic polymorphisms. *J Biol Chem* 1994; 269(32): 20256–20262.

15. Rousselle P, Keene DR, Ruggiero F, Champliaud MF, Rest M, and Burgeson RE. Laminin 5 binds the NC-1 domain of type VII collagen. *Journal of Cell Biology J Cell Biol* 1997; 138(3): 719–728.

16. Chen M, Marinkovich M, Veis A, Cai X, Rao C, O'Toole E, et al. Interactions of the amino-terminal noncollagenous (NC1) domain of type VII collagen with extracellular matrix components. A potential role in epidermal-dermal adherence in human skin. *J Biol Chem* 1997; 272(23): 14516–14522.

17. Rattenholl A, Pappano WN, Koch M, Keene DR, Kadler KE, Sasaki T, et al. Proteinases of the bone morphogenetic protein-1 family convert procollagen VII to mature anchoring fibril collagen. *J Biol Chem* 2002; 277(29): 26372–26378.

18. Yan EG, Paris JJ, Ahluwalia J, Lane AT, and Bruckner AL. Treatment decision-making for patients with the Herlitz subtype of junctional epidermolysis bullosa. *J Perinatol* 2007; 27(5): 307–311.

19. Yuen WY, Duipmans JC, Molenbuur B, Herpertz I, Mandema JM, and Jonkman MF. Long-term follow-up of patients with Herlitz-type junctional epidermolysis bullosa. *Br J Dermatol* 2012; 167(2): 374–382.

20. Ida JB, Livshitz I, Azizkhan RG, Lucky AW, and Elluru RG. Upper airway complications of junctional epidermolysis bullosa. *J Pediatr* 2012; 160(4): 657–661.

21. Has C, Bauer JW, Bodemer C, Bolling MC, Bruckner-Tuderman L, Diem A, et al. Consensus reclassification of inherited epidermolysis bullosa and other disorders with skin fragility. *British Journal of Dermatology* 2020: 1–14.

22. Eichstadt S, Tang JY, Solis DC, Siprashvili Z, Marinkovich MP, Whitehead N, et al. From clinical phenotype to genotypic modelling: Incidence and prevalence of recessive dystrophic epidermolysis bullosa (RDEB). *Clin Cosmet Investig Dermatol* 2019; 12: 933–942.

23. Has C, Nystrom A, Saeidian AH, Bruckner-Tuderman L, Uitto J. Epidermolysis bullosa: Molecular pathology of connective tissue components in the cutaneous basement membrane zone. *Matrix Biol* 2018; 71–72: 313–329.

24. Fine JD, Johnson LB, Weiner M, Li KP, and Suchindran C. Epidermolysis bullosa and the risk of life-threatening cancers: The national EB registry experience, 1986–2006. *J Am Acad Dermatol* 2009; 60(2): 203–211.

25. Hirsch T, Rothoeft T, Teig N, Bauer JW, Pellegrini G, De Rosa L, et al. Regeneration of the entire human epidermis using transgenic stem cells. *Nature* 2017; 551(7680): 327–332.

26. De Rosa L, Carulli S, Cocchiarella F, Quaglino D, Enzo E, Franchini E, et al. Long-term stability and safety of transgenic cultured epidermal stem cells in gene therapy of junctional epidermolysis bullosa. *Stem Cell Reports* 2014; 2(1): 1–8.

27. Rousselle P, Lunstrum GP, Keene DR, Burgeson RE. Kalinin: An epithelium-specific basement membrane adhesion molecule that is a component of anchoring filaments. *J Cell Biol* 1991; 114: 567–5676.

28. Sakai N, Waterman EA, Nguyen NT, Keene DR, and Marinkovich MP. Observations of skin grafts derived from keratinocytes expressing selectively engineered mutant laminin-332 molecules. *J Invest Dermatol* 2010; 130(8): 2147–2150.

29. Lazarova Z, Yee C, Darling T, Briggaman RA, and Yancey KB. Passive transfer of anti-laminin 5 antibodies induces subepidermal blisters in neonatal mice. *J Clin Invest* 1996; 98(7): 1509–1518.

30. De Rosa L, Secone Seconetti A, De Santis G, Pellacani G, Hirsch T, Rothoeft T, et al. Laminin 332-dependent YAP dysregulation depletes epidermal stem cells in junctional epidermolysis bullosa. *Cell Rep* 2019; 27(7): 2036–2049.

31. Siprashvili Z, Nguyen NT, Bezchinsky MY, Marinkovich MP, Lane AT, and Khavari PA. Long-term type VII collagen restoration to human epidermolysis bullosa skin tissue. *Hum Gene Ther* 2010; 21(10): 1299–1310.

32. Eichstadt S, Barriga M, Ponakala A, Teng C, Nguyen NT, Siprashvili Z, et al. Phase 1/2a clinical trial of gene-corrected autologous cell therapy for recessive dystrophic epidermolysis bullosa. *JCI Insight* 2019; 4(19).

33. Siprashvili Z, Nguyen NT, Gorell ES, Loutit K, Khuu P, Furukawa LK, et al. Safety and wound outcomes following genetically corrected autologous epidermal grafts in patients with recessive dystrophic epidermolysis bullosa. *JAMA—Journal of the American Medical Association* 2016; 316(17): 1808–1817.

34. Supp DM, Hahn JM, Combs KA, McFarland KL, Schwentker A, Boissy RE, et al. Collagen VII expression is required in both keratinocytes and fibroblasts for anchoring fibril formation in bilayer engineered skin substitutes. *Cell Transplant* 2019: 963689719857657.

35. Goto M, Sawamura D, Ito K, Abe M, Nishie W, Sakai K, et al. Fibroblasts show more potential as target cells than keratinocytes in COL7A1 gene therapy of dystrophic epidermolysis bullosa. *J Invest Dermatol* 2006; 126(4): 766–772.

36. Ortiz-Urda S, Lin Q, Green CL, Keene DR, Marinkovich MP, and Khavari PA. Injection of genetically engineered fibroblasts corrects regenerated human epidermolysis bullosa skin tissue. *J Clin Invest* 2003; 111(2): 251–255.

37. Georgiadis C, Syed F, Petrova A, Abdul-Wahab A, Lwin SM, Farzaneh F, et al. Lentiviral engineered fibroblasts expressing codon-optimized COL7A1 restore anchoring fibrils in RDEB. *Journal of Investigative Dermatology* 2016; 136(1): 284–292.

38. Lwin SM, Syed F, Di WL, Kadiyirire T, Liu L, Guy A, et al. Safety and early efficacy outcomes for lentiviral fibroblast gene therapy in recessive dystrophic epidermolysis bullosa. *JCI Insight* 2019; 4(11).

39. Marinkovich M, Lane A, Sridhar K, Keene D, Malyala A, and Maslowski J. A phase 1/2 study of genetically-corrected, collagen VII expressing autologous human dermal fibroblasts injected into the skin of patients with recessive dystrophic epidermolysis bullosa (RDEB). *Journal of Investigative Dermatology* 2018; 138(5): S100.

40. Marinkovich MP, Tang JY. Gene therapy for epidermolysis bullosa. *Journal of Investigative Dermatology* 2019; 139(6): 1221–1226.
41. Waterman EA, Sakai N, Nguyen NT, Horst BA, Veitch DP, Dey CN, et al. A laminin-collagen complex drives human epidermal carcinogenesis through phosphoinositol-3-kinase activation. *Cancer Res* 2007; 67(9): 4264–4270.
42. Mavilio F, Pellegrini G, Ferrari S, Di Nunzio F, Di Iorio E, Recchia A, et al. Correction of junctional epidermolysis bullosa by transplantation of genetically modified epidermal stem cells. *Nat Med* 2006; 12(12): 1397–1402.
43. Domloge-Hultsch N, Gammon WR, Briggaman RA, Gil SG, Carter WG, and Yancey KB. Epiligrin, the major human keratinocyte integrin ligand, is a target in both an acquired autoimmune and an inherited subepidermal blistering skin disease. *J Clin Invest* 1992; 90(4): 1628–1633.
44. Kirtschig G, Marinkovich MP, Burgeson RE, and Yancey KB. Anti-basement membrane autoantibodies in patients with anti-epiligrin cicatricial pemphigoid bind a subunit of laminin 5. *J Invest Dermatol* 1995; 105(4): 543–548.
45. Ortiz-Urda S, Garcia J, Green CL, Chen L, Lin Q, Veitch DP, et al. Type VII collagen is required for Ras-driven human epidermal tumorigenesis. *Science* 2005; 307(5716): 1773–1776.
46. Woodley DT, Burgeson RE, Lunstrum G, Bruckner-Tuderman L, Reese MJ, Briggaman RA. Epidermolysis bullosa acquisita antigen is the globular carboxyl terminus of type VII procollagen. *J Clin Invest* 1988; 81(3): 683–687.
47. Hacein-Bey-Abina S, Von Kalle C, Schmidt M, McCormack MP, Wulffraat N, Leboulch P, et al. LMO2-associated clonal T cell proliferation in two patients after gene therapy for SCID-X1. *Science* 2003; 302(5644): 415–459.
48. Hacein-Bey-Abina S, von Kalle C, Schmidt M, Le Deist F, Wulffraat N, McIntyre E, et al. A serious adverse event after successful gene therapy for X-linked severe combined immunodeficiency. *N Engl J Med* 2003; 348(3): 255–256.
49. Dunbar CE, High KA, Joung JK, Kohn DB, Ozawa K, and Sadelain M. Gene therapy comes of age. *Science* 2018; 359(6372).

Precision CAR-T Cell Therapy for Autoimmune Blistering Diseases

11

Lawrence S. Chan

Contents

INTRODUCTION

Chimeric antigen receptor T cell therapy (CAR-T cell therapy) a like a "living drug" that utilizes a patient's own immune cells (T cell, T lymphocyte) to do the therapeutic action, after they are modified in a laboratory setting [1, 2]. The

DOI: 10.1201/9781003121275-15

original idea of this therapy is deduced from the possibility that cancer-specific T cells could eradicate tumors [3]. This therapeutic method takes advantage of the knowledge that genetically modified T cells can eliminate the target cell by interacting with the target cell in a MHC-nonrestricted manner. The early CAR-T cell therapies were developed to target cancers, particularly to those B cell hematologic malignancies that occur during childhood. Some of the early successes of CAR-T cell treatment include a CD19-targeted therapy and a CD22-targeted therapy for acute lymphocytic lymphoma of B-cell origin, with complete elimination of those B cell lymphomas [4–6]. As an adaptive immunotherapy, the CAR-T cell method involves three major steps [1]:

- Patient's peripheral blood is collected and their T cells isolated.
- These isolated T cells will be modified with genetic engineering technique *ex vivo* in a sterile laboratory setting. As a result of this modification, these bioengineered T cells will carry a chimeric antigen receptor on their surface linked with a co-stimulatory molecule in the cytoplasm, ready to recognize their designated target on the surface of B-origin lymphoma cells and cause cytolysis (cell destruction) of the target B cells. In one study, these T cells were bioengineered to carry a single chain of antibody variable region recognizing CD19, a surface marker of B cell lineage. These engineered T cells thus were able to bind to B cells and induce cytolysis.
- These modified T cells are then activated in the laboratory and reintroduced into patient's blood to fight the targeted B-origin lymphoma cells.

The recent success of CAR-T cell therapies on human neoplastic diseases subsequently led to the idea that this method of treatment could be modified and utilized to manage autoimmune diseases that are mediated by autoimmune B lymphocytes [2, 7].

ANALYSIS OF THE NEED

Autoimmune diseases are mediated by the patient's altered immune system against their own cells, tissues, or organs, resulting in organ dysfunction and destruction. The life-altering impact of autoimmune disease is keenly stated by Joan Friedlander: "As with many life-altering events, an autoimmune illness is almost guaranteed to cause you to re-evaluate your priorities" [8]. Although each autoimmune disease entity is relatively rare, collectively, as a group of more than 80 entities, they become one of the most prevalent diseases, affecting between 14 and 23 million people in the US alone. It is estimated that the annual direct healthcare costs for autoimmune diseases in the US amounts to $100 billion [9]. Because the significant impact of autoimmune disease on society, the National Institutes of Health in the US spent more than $590 million for research on autoimmune diseases in fiscal year 2003 alone [10]. Autoimmune skin diseases can be mediated by autoreactive T cells or autoantibodies. This chapter will focus on one of the skin diseases caused by autoantibodies, those mediated by autoimmune B cells. The most common entities of this group of diseases are two autoimmune blistering diseases—pemphigus vulgaris and bullous pemphigoid—which are targeted by autoantibodies against epidermal cell surface components and epidermal-dermal junction components, respectively [11–13]. While bullous pemphigoid is commonly controlled by low doses of immunosuppressives and corticosteroids, pemphigus vulgaris is known to be resistant to conventional treatments and is life threatening. Hence, pemphigus vulgaris is the primary focus of this chapter.

Pemphigus vulgaris is manifested clinically as a superficial blistering disease. In a majority of patients, the clinical presentation is initially observed within the oral cavity, with erythema, blisters, and erosions. These oral lesions are typically painful and substantially interfere patient's food and fluid intake. When skin surface is involved, it typically affects any part of the skin, including the scalp, face, trunk, extremities, and other mucosal surfaces. The blisters are usually flaccid and easily broken, leaving behind many erosions, thus leading to fluid and electrolyte loss and the possibility of infection. Besides its typical clinical presentation, the diagnosis of pemphigus vulgaris is generally confirmed by the results of examination of a lesional skin biopsy and a peri-lesional skin biopsy. While the lesional skin obtained from these patients will show a characteristic intra-epidermal blister with acantholysis (epidermal cell-cell separation) and inflammatory cell infiltration, peri-lesional skin specimens that are processed for direct immunofluorescence microscopy will reveal IgG and C3 autoantibodies binding the epidermal cell surfaces in a net-like pattern. Additional diagnostic studies, including indirect immunofluorescence microscopy and ELISA, can be performed to further certify the disease diagnosis and assess the extent of disease-causing antibodies through their titer determination. While an indirect immunofluorescence study on monkey esophagus epithelium substrate commonly reveals the patient's presence and quantity of the circulating IgG class of autoantibodies binding epithelial cell surfaces in a net-like pattern, ELISA usually confirms the patient's circulating IgG autoantibodies, specifically recognizing desmogleins 3 and 1 antigens at the molecular level [11, 12]. Studies have pointed out that autoantibodies targeting desmoglein 1 and desmoglein 3 are responsible for the occurrence of blisters in the skin and the mucosae, respectively [13, 14].

Although the diagnosis of pemphigus vulgaris is usually straightforward, the treatment is a totally different story. The treatments for patients affected by pemphigus vulgaris have gone through several major historic phases of evolution. Before the development of systemic corticosteroids as a therapeutic medication, patients suffering from this disease generally received supportive treatment only, and most patients died from this disease during this time frame of first treatment phase. During the time of the second historic treatment phase, when systemic corticosteroid became available and was utilized for these patients' treatment, many patients survived the disease, but the life-saving medication inevitably resulted in severe side effects from long-term use: diabetes, cataracts, osteopathy, and substantial weight gain. In the next treatment phase, physicians gained the knowledge of general immunosuppressives and utilized them to partially substitute for systemic corticosteroid, thereby reducing the quantity and duration of systemic steroid usage and decreasing the steroid-related side effects. However, the negative aspect of these non-specific immunosuppressives would have potentially dangerous suppressive effects on the patients' overall immune defense against pathogens and open the door for serious opportunistic infections [12]. This brings us to the fourth and current phase of treatment, which was initiated around 2006, when a biologic medication termed rituximab became the treatment choice for many patients [15, 16]. Rituximab is a monoclonal antibody targeting a middle development stage of human B cells—those cells that possess cell surface marker CD20—before they became committed antibody-producing plasma cells and lost the CD20 marker [2]. Rituximab, a chimeric antibody that fuses a human CD20-binding mouse variable region (Fv) and a human constant (Fc) region, has offered patients a better treatment option, as it will target only the B-cell arm of the immune defense and thus will be less of a problem in generating a general immunosuppression in the patients because it does not affect T cell immunity in any significant way. Mechanistically, rituximab depletes B cells by binding to CD20, followed by depleting CD20+ B cells through one of the four possible ways that have been clearly defined: complement-dependent cytotoxicity, antibody-dependent cytotoxicity, antibody-dependent phagocytosis, and induction of programmed cell death (apoptosis). The depletion of B cells then results in general reduction of antibody production, including the pathogenic antibodies targeting desmogleins [2]. Although rituximab is highly effective and provides a good treatment option, it is not a precision therapy that would target only those pathogenic B cells. As the medical community continue to seek a more perfect solution in managing pemphigus vulgaris, CAR-T cell-directed therapy responds to the challenge, and this potential therapeutic option will be detailed in the paragraphs that follow.

THE TECHNOLOGY: CAR-T CELL TREATMENT FOR PEMPHIGUS VULGARIS

The recent development of CAR-T cell-directed therapy has brought lots of excitement to physicians who care for patients with autoimmune skin diseases and scientists who study autoimmunity of the skin. A group of researchers have generated a chimeric autoantibody receptor (CAAR)-T cell methodology, aiming to develop a novel and target-specific treatment for pemphigus vulgaris. The invention of this method is based on the knowledge that the pathogenic B cells in pemphigus vulgaris bear a cell membrane–found anti-desmoglein 3 autoantibody as their B cell receptors and the theory that T cells engineered to contain receptors specific for these pathogenic B cells can induce cytolysis of these B cells. In this case, "AA" or autoantibody is equivalent to the "antigen" in the CAR designation [17], and the "AAR" or autoantibody receptor in the bioengineered CAAR-T cell will be constructed to bear the segment of desmoglein 3 protein that is the receptor for the anti-desmoglein 3 autoantibody on the B cell receptor of pathogenic B cell surfaces. Some details of this interesting study are described next.

- The researchers performed cloning of the gene encoding fusion protein CAAR, comprising three domains: an extracellular domain of human desmoglein 3 fragment, which serves as anti-demoglein 3 autoantibody recognition domain; a transmembrane domain; and an intracellular domain that contains two parts: the zeta (ζ) chain of CD3 (a component of endogenous T-cell receptor) and co-stimulatory molecules (4–1BB/CD137) for promotion of survival and proliferation purposes. In this study, experimentally determined to be most potent in cytolysis of B cells bearing anti-desmoglein 3 receptors, the CAAR portion is composed of extracellular cadherin domains 1–4 (EC1–4) of desmoglein 3, the dimerization-competent CD8a transmembrane domain, and CD137-CD3ζ cytoplasmic domain.
- Cloned the CAAR gene into lentiviral plasmids.
- Transfected the CAAR-containing viral vectors into packaging cell line to obtain sufficient quantity of CAAR-bearing plasmids.
- Mouse T cells were collected and isolated from the same strain of mice affected by pemphigus vulgaris.
- Incubated the isolated T cells with CAAR-bearing plasmids to allow these plasmids to enter the T cells and introduce the CAAR-encoding RNA to these T cells.

- The CAAR RNA was reversely transcribed to DNA and integrated into the genomes of these T cells.
- These bioengineered T cells transcribed and translated the CAAR gene and expressed CAAR proteins on their cell surfaces.
- These CAAR-T cells were activated, expanded, concentrated, and cryopreserved *ex vivo*.
- The functions of these CAAR-T cells in cytolysis of pathogenic B cells were examined *in vitro*.
- These CAAR-T cells, confirmed to be functional *in vitro*, were reinfused into the mouse with disease caused by anti-human desmoglein 3 autoantibodies. A schematic diagram depicts the structure of the CAAR-T cell, its binding interaction with the anti-desmoglein-bearing pathogenic B cell, and the possible mechanism of subsequent B cell cytolysis in Figure 11.1.

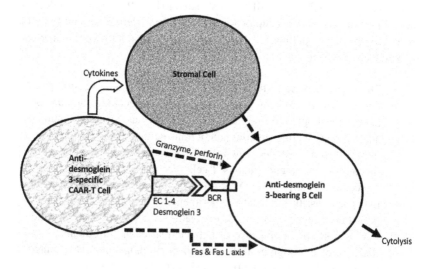

FIGURE 11.1 The binding of CAAR-T cell to anti-desmoglein-bearing B cell and the possible cytolytic mechanisms. The binding is established between the EC1–4 domain of desmoglein 3 protein on the CAAR-T cell receptor and the anti-desmoglein 3 on the B cell receptor. The cytolysis of anti-desmoglein 3–bearing B cells is possibly carried out by one of the three mechanisms: direct cytolysis through granzyme and perforin, apoptosis via Fas and Fas L axis, or indirect cytolysis by cytokine-induced activation of stromal cells.

Some of the interesting findings from this study are [17]:

- These CAAR-T cells selectively targeted human anti-desmoglein 3–bearing B cells *in vitro* and were able to target those pathogenic B cells bearing antibodies against different epitopes of human desmoglein 3.
- Human patients' anti-desmoglein 3 autoantibodies did decrease but did not hinder the cytotoxic activity of these CAAR-T cells *in vitro*.
- In a mouse model of pemphigus vulgaris induced by autoantibodies to human desmoglein 3, these CAAR-T cells reduced pathogenic IgG antibodies and decreased the clinical disease severity.
- Off-target toxicity against keratinocytes, which express desmocollin and other desmoglein protein that could theoretically bind to the desmoglein 3 of the CAAR-T cells and become unintended targets, was not observed.
- These CAAR-T cells that specifically target anti-desmoglein B cells had similar targeting activity to non-specific CD19-target CAR-T cells, suggesting no reduction of efficacy when these CAAR-T cells target self-reactive B cells.

The same group of researchers recently reported the following findings of a preclinical study: Desmoglein 3-CAAR T cells specifically lysed human anti-desmoglein 3 B cells derived from human pemphigus vulgaris patients, reduced circulating and in-situ bound autoantibodies, and cleared blisters on clinical and histological levels [18].

UNFINISHED BUSINESS

Before CAAR-T cell therapy becomes a standard treatment option for patients affected by pemphigus vulgaris, a few issues need to be resolved.

Targeting Anti-Desmoglein 1–Bearing B Cells

For most patients with pemphigus vulgaris, for whom the initial disease manifested inside their oral mucous membranes and who have autoantibodies to desmoglein 3, their subsequent disease involvement in the skin location is marked by the surface of additional autoantibodies to desmoglein 1 as well

[13, 14]. This observation strongly suggests that for those patients manifesting both mucosal and skin diseases, we will need CAAR-T cells to target anti-desmoglein 1–bearing B cells as well as CAAR-T cells targeting anti-desmoglein 3–bearing B cells, if our goal is to achieve complete disease control for pemphiugus vulgaris [2]. Anti-desmoglein 1–specific CAAR-T cells will also be a perfect living medication to treat patients affected by pemphigus foliaceus, which is mediated by autoantibodies to desmoglein 1 only [13, 14].

Establishing Treatment Schedule

Another issue the medical community needs to settle is how often we need to provide CAAR-T cell therapy for a given patient. Although there are suggestions that some of the bioengineered CAAR-T cells may become memory T cells and therefore would provide permanent protection to prevent disease relapse from resurgence of anti-desmoglein-bearing pathogenic B cells, we will be better served if such evidence is documented in real-life patients. This treatment schedule is important to establish in light of the prohibitive cost of this living medication, as a single dose of CD19-specific CAR-T cell treatment for hematologic B cell lymphoma costs approximately $40,000 [2]. Furthermore, patients who relapsed and required additional treatment have been documented in CAR-T cell therapy of CD19-specific B cell lymphomas [3].

Relapse Management

The initial success of CD19-specific CAR-T cell therapy for hematologic B cell lymphoma was hindered by a lack of long-term remission in some patients, as relapsed cases surfaced. Most often, the reason was the loss of antigen (CD19) in B cell tumors. Prospective anticipation of potential antigen loss could help in setting up a strategy to encounter these possible long-term treatment failures, as additional CD22-specific CAR-T cells were used successfully to counter the relapse from CD19-specific CAR-T cell therapy [4].

Further Understanding

In CAR-T cell therapy for B lymphoma, it is generally understood that CAR-T cells can initiate B cell tumor cytolysis using three possible mechanisms [3]:

- Utilize the granzyme and perforin axis to lysis antigen-positive B cell tumors.

- Utilize the Fas and FasL pathway to target antigen-negative portion of B cell tumors within the antigen-positive milieu.
- Utilize cytokines to upregulate IFN-γ receptors on nearby stromal cells, thereby facilitating stromal cell attack on B lymphoma cells.

At this juncture, our understanding of the detailed mechanism and adverse effects of CAR-T cell is still limited. Therefore, we need to conduct more studies to delineate relevant information for the medical community to develop optimal therapeutic plans and to minimize serious adverse effects [3].

SUMMARY

The medical advancement of CAR-T cell therapy for B cell–mediated disease opens the door for potential treatment of autoimmune blistering skin diseases. It is hoped that further search in this area will bear fruit for a more precise target-specific management for this group of diseases.

REFERENCES

1. Chan LS. Precision. In: Chan LS and Tang WC. Eds. *Engineering-Medicine: Principles and Applications of Engineering in Medicine.* CRC Press, Boca Raton, FL, 2019.
2. Didona D, Maglie R, Eming R, et al. Pemphigus: Current and future therapeutic strategies. *Front Immunol* 2019; June 25. Doi: 10.3389/fimmu.2019.01418.
3. Benmebarek M-R, Karches CH, Cadilha BL, et al. Killing mechanisms of chimeric antigen receptor (CAR) T cells. *Int J Mol Sci* 2019; 20: 1283. Doi: 10.3390/ijms20061283.po.
4. Kochenderfer JN, Wilson WH, Janik JE, et al. Eradication of B-lineage cells and regression of lymphoma in a patient treated with autologous T cells genetically engineered to recognize CD19. *Blood* 2010: 4099–4102.
5. MacKall CL, Merchant MS, and Fry TJ. Immune based therapies for childhood cancer. *Nature Review Clinical Oncology* 2014; 11: 693–703.
6. Fry TJ, Shah NN, Orentas RJ, et al. CD22-targeted CAR-T cells induced remission in B-ALL that is naïve or resistant to CD19-targeted CAR immunotherapy. *Nat Med* 2018; 24: 20–28.
7. Chatenould L. Precision medicine for autoimmune disease. *Nat Biotechnol* 2016; 34: 930–932. Doi: 10.1038/nbt.3670.
8. [GOODREADS] Autoimmune disease quotes. Goodreads. [www.goodreads/tag/autoimmune-disease] Accessed December 19, 2020.

9. Beecham JE and Seneff S. Autoimmune disease: Budget-buster or enlightened solutions? (The coming epidemic and the new administration in Washington). *Arch Comm Med and Pub Health* 2017; 3: 032–040. http:/dx.doi.org/10.17352/2455-5479.000022.

10. [PROGRESS] Progress in autoimmune diseases research. Report to congress. National Institutes of Health. March 2005. [www.niaid.nih.gov/sites/default/files/adccfinal.pdf] Accessed December 26, 2020.

11. Chan LS. *Blistering skin diseases.* CRC Press, Boca Raton, FL, 2009.

12. Chan LS. *Pemphigus vulgaris.* Nova Science Publisher, Hauppauge, NY, 2016.

13. Kasperkiewicz M, Ellebrecht CT, Takahashi H, et al. Pemphigus. *Nat Rev Dis Primers* 2018; 3: 17026. Doi: 10.1038/nrdp.2017.26.

14. Mahoney MG, Wang Z, Rothenberger K, et al. Explanations for the clinical and microscopic localization of lesions in pemphigus foliaceus and vulgaris. *J Clin Invest* 1999; 103: 461–468.

15. Ahmed AR, Spigelman Z, Cavacini LA, et al. Treatment of pemphigus vulgaris with rituximab and intravenous immune globulin. *N Engl J Med* 2006; 355U: 1772–1779. Doi: 10.1056/NEJMoa062930.

16. Joly P, Mouquet H, Roujeau JC, et al. A single cycle of rituximab for the treatment of severe pemphigus. *N Engl J Med* 2007; 357: 545–552. Doi: 10.1056/NEJMoa067752.

17. Ellebrecht CT, Bhoj VG, Nace A, et al. Reengineering chimeric antigen receptor T cells for targeted therapy of autoimmune disease. *Science* 2016; 353: 179–184. Doi: 10.1126/science.aaf6756.

18. Lee J, Lundgren DK, Mao X, et al. Antigen-specific B cell depletion for precision therapy of mucosal pemphigus vulgaris. *J Clin Invest* 2020; 130: 6317–6324. Doi: 10.1172/JCI138416.

Index

Note: Numbers in *italic* indicate a figure on the corresponding page.